# Flirt Diva

*FOR SINGLE WOMEN WHO WANT TO HAVE A FABULOUS LIFE!*

*Sue Ostler*

*Your 6-Week-Plan To Get Loved Up*

Published in the UK by MX Publishing
ISBN 9781904312796

335 Princess Park Manor, Royal Drive,
London, N11 3GX
www.mxpublishing.co.uk

Cover Design by Staunch Design
www.staunch.com

**Warning!**

*ONLY READ THIS IF YOU ARE PREPARED TO BE RESPONSIBLE FOR HIGH VOLTAGE ROCK 'N' ROLL SEXUAL CHEMISTRY!*

## About the author

Dubbed the Flirt Diva by the *Metro* UK and Queen of Love by *New Woman* magazine, Sue has been a recognised spokesperson in the field of dating and relationships since launching *Vodka & Chocolate Love Therapy* in 2004.

Sue's undying belief that there's a Flirt Diva in every woman just waiting to burst out, has fuelled a unique collaboration with all things flirting.

In 2008, Sue created her alter ego, the wildly saucy, outspoken, Flirt Diva, star of the travelling Vodka & Chocolate Flirt-Shows, and host of a gaggle of girly nights from Flirting & Burlesquing Hour; Flirt n' Throb Hula-Hoop parties; and of course, The Great Big Vodka & Chocolate, Cocktail and Cupcake Afternoon Tease Parties. Guaranteed to leave you feeling deliciously, decadently feminine - and just a little bit naughty...Find out more at: www.flirtdiva.com

**Sue's previous books: The *Get Over It!* Series:**
*Get Over It! Allen & Unwin1998*
*Get On With It! Allen & Unwin 2002*
*Relationships that Rock! Allen & Unwin 2003*

To Edward Lee. Thank you.

And especially to my mum and dad for encouraging me follow my dreams.
This book is for you.

## Acknowledgments

Thanks to Jessica Ainscough, contributing editor; Katerina Georgiou, quiz maestro; Celia Morgan, creative whiz and events queen; Ravneet Ahluwalia, for editing and proofing; Anita Carroll, make-up queen; Jessica Adams for her ongoing support; Angie Kuzma for the boozy marketing pow-wows; Danielle Waller, Speeddater queen; Ann and Ryan at www.metro.co.uk; the Benefit Cosmetics gals; Renee at the Women's Erotic Emporium; Memo at the Cupcake Emporium, Simon at LateNightLondon; Alexi Duggins, Joly Braime and the rest of the original Itchy crew.
Special thanks to all the girls who've supported me throughout this crazy Vodka & Chocolate journey.
And especially to my mum and dad for letting me follow my dreams.

Starting a new life in a new country is never easy – but you guys made it rock.
Thank you!

***Why flirting is better than sex:***

- *You can GET flirting*

- *Flirting satisfies – even when it's all over*

- *You can flirt safely while you are driving*

- *You can make a flirtation last as long as you want it to*

- *You can flirt in front of your mother*

- *A good flirt won't make him want to go sleep afterwards*

- *The word "commitment" doesn't scare off flirts*

- *With flirting there's no need to fake it*

- *Flirting won't make you pregnant*

- *You can have a flirt any time of the month*

- *Good flirts are easy to find*

- *You can have as many kinds of flirtations as you can handle*

- *You are never too young or too old for flirting*

- *Flirting doesn't keep your neighbors awake*

- *Flirting won't give you an STD*

- *With flirting, size doesn't matter*

### *The Flirt Diva-ography*

Once upon a time, this Flirt Diva made a vow to flirt. I became the Bridezilla of flirting. I was flirting's most passionate disciple. My calling began many moons ago and since then I've immersed myself in it. Now I'm sharing the secrets with you – because everyone knows that life's more fun when you're a fully divafied Flirt Diva.

Whichever way you look at it, I am a flirt. And sure there have been times when I've lost my nerve, fluffed my lines and walked away when I should have stayed and played. But hey, I'm not perfect. I just love flirting and I'll tell you why – it makes me feel indestructible. I've been doing it for a long time and it still happens with eye-popping regularity.

I may be happily loved up in a long-term relationship, but you don't hear me complain when the hottie at my local bookshop showers me with undivided attention, I just beam mischievously and reward him with a smile and an eyelash shimmy. It's taken a lifetime of practice, but like the best things, the ability to flirt just gets better. It's like being in love. I like that too. What's not to love? Regular sex, champagne cocktails, candle-lit dinners and – marriage proposals.

I'm not talking out of school when I tell you I've had my share of proposals – even from the rich and the famous. John Cleese asked me to marry him once (he claims he was joking, but so what? He still asked.) And those propositions and declarations of love you'll read about in the pages to come, they're legit. And really, who hasn't been hit on by a world famous rock star? Oops, mustn't kiss and tell. So many admirers, so little time.

Look at all my proposals, poems and flirt-o-grams. Here's one from Tom. Here's one from Dick. Here's one from Harry. I would have been married three times by now, if I'd said yes every time a proposal came along, but it wasn't my choice. That's because I understand a husband is for ever, not just Christmas.

"How?" My girlfriends ask suspiciously, "Do you do it?"

Easy.

A shimmy here, a slither there, a slinky everywhere. I've never thought twice about making an excuse to sashay in a littler closer, or stroke someone's shoulder to make my point. To clasp another's forearms while I kiss their cheek, and cup their hand while getting a cigarette light; to lower my eyelids, purse my lips; to linger and lock eyes over a handshake, or use my voice to create that intimate *"it's just and you and me"* vibe.

I'm a fan of the slow burn, which doesn't scream as much as whisper just a *hint* of what's to come. But that's not all, I know how to transmit a bold signal with a well-timed touch, to thrust out a cocky wink and make eyes at a beautiful stranger across a crowded room.

I might like talking, but I *love* listening, and it's a well-known fact that listening is the most seductive thing in the world. So you see there's nothing sexually brash about this approach – it's just me. I'm warm. I'm friendly. I'm natural, I'm approachable. Hey I'm a middle child, I need the attention!

My flirtosophy has never been limited by dreary details like age, circumstance or personality. I've flirted for love, lust, friendship and random acts of kindness, as much I've flirted in the interest of a better quality of life. It makes me feel alive and hopefully makes others feels great too.

You have a lot of gumption, one of my disciples said.

No shit.

But look, don't get me wrong. If you were to see me in action, you wouldn't think it was some spoof from a *Carry On* film. It's not like I fling

9

myself into lust overdrive, hurtling and hip-shaking my way around the place. I don't throw out shag-me-senseless-smiles, or cause jaws to hit the floor while I gush about the benefits of the Anne Summers dominatrix kit for beginners. It's ah, more subtle.

I've never known flirting to be anything but harmless. That's because it's always been well-intentioned and low key. I've never flirted for intent, as much as I've flirted for fun. It's my way of communicating: an instinctive, genuine reflex backed up by a big, breezy smile.

Which is why I've decided to share a warts-and-all snapshot from my Flirt Diva vault. I'm willing to do this for one reason only. If you truly want to transform yourself into a killer flirt, you'll need to know a whole lot more than how to send your message with a saucy well-timed wink and a game of touchy-feelies.

You will need to go back in time and remember the first time you flirted. How did it feel? How did you react? Can you recall that explosive flash when you first became sexually aware, or the erotic shock of your earliest ever sexual jolt? That "A-ha!" moment where you recognised the signals you were getting were driven by pure hurdy-gurdy-flirty-dirty lust? How did you know when someone was sexually interested in you? Did you blush like a little pink cocktail sausage? I know I did!

Soon I'll ask you to have a go at reconstructing your own personal history. You'll get started at the end of Step 1 where you'll find details on how to record your own personal Love CV. Once you've got the ball rolling, keep jotting down the juicy stuff as it comes to you. Meanwhile, here's a tiny snippet from my Love CV.

So, there I was, a 30-something Bridget Jones singleton. Was I a new breed of woman who chose freedom? Or was I single simply because I hadn't met The One? Whichever it was, I was keen to keep looking. So I decided to take a long overdue break from the sometimes exhausting world of relationships and get out there and road-test the realms of flirting material I'd picked up during my lifelong love odyssey.

I was ready to swash-buckle my way across a wild stormy sea of dark-eyed, dashing men; all of who would be intoxicated by the sheer force of my personality. Before they knew what had hit them, they'd have fallen madly, badly in lust with me (in my dreams anyway). I was ripe for this. Ready to be ravished. It was time to have some fun and put the glint in my eye to the test. In return I would be the happiest most loved-up Flirt Diva I could be. And who knows, maybe I'd meet Captain Marvellous along the way.

I knew only too well what it was like going through the token single phase. It can drag on for longer than planned – it could be months, or it could be years. I got to the point where I'd just had enough of being single. I was going on my route to work and back again every freakin' day.
I never looked left or right, just straight ahead. I was living my life in tunnel vision. I knew I had to open my eyes and look around. I had to gather my wits and have the guts to be direct. I had to stop the games and lay it on the line. I had to reinvent myself. So I did.

I bought myself a hula hoop and made a sequinned headband. I used a cigarette holder and pinned flowers in my hair. I learnt belly dancing and took burlesque lessons and went to classes for bubbled buttocks and troubled tums. I ate toasted love-muffins and wore long satin gloves and cherry patent heels. I went to fancy-dress parties in a beehive wig and lashings of 60s eyeliner. I laughed in the face of dowdy fashion, party poopers and ignorant men. I propelled myself right out of my comfort zone. And pretty soon I got myself a boyfriend. A few years in the love bubble later, and I'm engaged to be married. How did I do it? I gave him a smile; sauntered over and I just worked that surgically attached wonder bra.

11

Seriously though, it wasn't just my saucy brand of sass that nailed it – though god knows it helped – it was more that I'd taken the time to figure stuff out. I knew what I wanted. I knew what had to be done. I had to put myself out there. So I just did it.

In the end I got my wish, and along the way I got much more than I ever bargained for. I won. I lost. I screwed up. I mislaid my dignity and encountered one or two of the truly bizarre situations I've ever known. But most importantly, I put myself out there and learnt by my mistakes and the mini trails of daredevil destruction I left behind. That's what made me the person I am today and inspired me to develop the Flirt Diva theory. It's what put me on this mission to get *you* loved up.

So now my little minxes and seductresses-in-training, I'm inviting you, as my always vamptastic VIP's to the world's first ever Flirt-Shimmy. Think of this as your own personal, sexy road-trip where together we will share sizzling secrets designed to get your head in the flirt zone.

Yes ladies, it's all about getting out there and trying your luck on the Wheel of Flirting Fortune. We're here because you want to be noticed. You want to turn heads and you want to be a walking, talking dynamo. So strap yourself into the Flirt Divamobile, and hang on for the ride as you relive the good, the bad and the ugly experiences that awakened your sexuality and shaped the Flirt Diva you are on your way to becoming.

♥          ♥          ♥

# How it Works!

Welcome to the world of the Flirt Diva! Here you'll find Vol.1 of all your flirty female superheroes rolled into one. It's everything you always wanted to know about flirting, but were too afraid to ask. We'll be studying the flirtabolical do's and don'ts, you'll learn how to read gestures and dish out cheeky banter, and pretty soon you'll have all the hallmarks of a warrior Flirt Diva as you hurtle and head-flick your way around life. This is your bible people.

You'll go behind the scenes with the Flirt Diva disciples where you'll stroke and poke, preen and pout, and move in closer with flying fingers that caress, dip and tease. Learn to mesmerise with your eyes not your thighs, naughty smirks and cheeky quirks. We'll be studying the theory as well as the practical – what to say and what to do. You don't have to be OTT and it doesn't matter how poor you think your game is, you can learn these skills. *And ssshhh! This is secret women's information!*

Along the way I'll dish the dirt on all things from sex and lust to the morning after pill. We'll play some Flirt Diva games, I'll reveal secrets of the Great Flirt Divas and tell you some bedtime stories. I'll share what I've learnt through my own personal experiences, not to mention the post break-up therapy – vodka therapy that is! Or at least what I can remember of it.

Keep in mind, the advice that follows will only be effective if you're gung-ho and prepared to take a risk. You will have to get out of your comfort zone. If that's you, and you're up for the challenge – take aim and get ready to flirt!

### *Tools and Rules*

Here's how the book works. There are two key tools which we'll use throughout to help find your flirting mojo. A proper super-flirt awakening requires the consistent use of both. Because, in order to unleash your inner Flirt Diva, first you need to find it!

There are 6-Steps which feature a Fill-Out-and-Keep Flirt-Plan and contain the 7-day challenges. You will work through the tasks as they occur and record the results in your Flirt Diary. You'll be doing the challenges over 6 consecutive weeks. Each task takes an average of 30 minutes and is done mainly from the safety of your own home, so no excuses!

Secondly, you will write up a Flirt Review at the completion of each step. This is where you record your thoughts in response to the challenges you've worked through. This is part of the procedure that will ultimately reveal your signature flirting style and help develop your profile. You may think you have very little to say on the subject, but once you've done a week's worth of exercises and you put pen to paper, you're likely to surprise yourself with all sorts of super-girl thoughts. You can put anything you like down on the page, it's all part of the work in process. So get yourself a pen, an A6 bound notebook, a sense of humour and settle in as we develop your personalised love program!

### *Flirt Gang Rules*

Did you ever do that thing, where it's just the two of you in a cosy candlelit cocktail bar and the "last drinks" bell has rung, and you want to turn things up a notch, so you put one hand on his thigh and the other on your car keys, raise your eyebrows suggestively and ask if he has, "any condoms?"

No, neither did I

But I have seen this kind of thing happen and let me say right here and now, these are not the antics of a Flirt Diva in training. I'm all for binge flirting, but not cringe flirting! Don't be going all OTT and acting like you're desperate to race him off into the night if that's not the message you want to put out there.

Of course it's the easiest thing in the world to make some random guy think you're the most luscious cherry cream-pie on the desert menu, but please refrain if you are not prepared to go home with him – and have sex. You don't want to be talked about as some come hither-and-dither prick-tease do you? And if there's one thing you will learn in the following flirt-opedia, it's that once you take that first step and commit to someone, you need to follow it though.

If you come across like a total floozy and give the impression you're up for sex, of course he'll try to drag you back to his cave! So don't act all coy and surprised when he does. And don't expect him to call when he says he will, if you *do* fall for it on the First Night. You need to make a pledge that from now on, you're going to be in control. You'll be calling the shots thanks very much.

### Take note

The subtext should never be "you're asking for it".

Flirting in the work place has dodgy connotations, so I'm not going there.

Flirting when you're off your face has dangerous connotations, so DON'T DO IT!

Know the difference between the tasteful, playful flirt and the obnoxious flirt.

Learn how to recognise the signs when someone is trying to tell you to "go away!"

This is not about dumbing yourself down to "get your way".

Know the difference between sexy and slutty.

Always be assertive, not aggressive.

Those who cross the line are Flirts Behaving Badly and they're not welcome here.

Negative flirts are heavy handed and they spoil the fun for everyone else.

Know your own limitations. Make your own guidelines. Use your head.

Don't flirt with sexual intent unless you want to end up in bed with the guy.

Flirt socially as though your life depends on it.
Don't live with regret, if there's someone you like, get on with it!

***Flirt Diva Checklist:***

- Confidence

- Intelligence

- Charm

- Sex appeal

- Saucy smile

- Sass

The benefit of the Get Loved Up! plan is that you can adapt it to any situation – romantic, social or professional – and it will *continue* to work for you long after you've finished reading. Along the way, you'll learn how to prepare for *anything* that comes your way.

Keep in mind that while flirting has the power to supercharge all aspects of your life and amp up your confidence, it doesn't necessarily come naturally. But the good news is – anyone can do it. All you need is a splash of the 3 P's – persistence, perseverance and if that fails – a personality transplant!

By the time you've finished filling in the blanks dedicated to getting loved up, you will be well and truly out of emotional rehab and set to enter the relationship bonanza. Ready to consolidate all the areas of your life so your career and social life work in harmony with your love life, *and not against it.* As you begin to move out of apathy mode and into passion mode, you'll be less likely to feel frustrated with the state of your romantic life, or the lack of it.

Think of this as your own personal love-in, where in addition to dedicating yourself to friends, fitness, socialising or career, you will start building the foundations for a sexy new life. Along the way you'll develop an alter ego who will let you be the confidence queen you've always dreamt of being. Think Beyoncés, Sasha Fierce stage creation – a dirty dancing fantasy figure who lets Beyoncé get away with the jaw-dropping porn-style moves that she couldn't otherwise. Having your own alter ego means you can get away with almost anything. And the fun starts here!

♥                    ♥                              ♥

# *Introduction*

Hello pussycats, let's talk about what you want, what you really, really want. Do you want to be noticed?  Do you want to be charismatic? Do you want to walk into the room and have heads turn?  If the answer is a high fivin' "Yes!" then keep on reading because the Flirt Diva is about to divulge all.

Every aspiring Flirt Diva knows how potent you can be when you approach life's challenges as a Triple S: a saucier, smarter, sassier version of yourself. But it's not just about flirting; it's about kicking butt as a woman. Whether you're a Prada obsessed party princess who thrives on a good time, but wouldn't recognise a flirt sign if it came up and hit you over the head; or you're a timid type who just wants advice on how to snare a snog – this is the book for you. But hey, I don't have to tell you that, you're a cluey miss, that's why you're here. You've already taken the first step. Now it's time to reignite your inner goddess and go for it.

But this is not about setting booby traps. The reason we're here is to sharpen our collective flirting skills, stay ahead in this fuzzy "anything goes" love climate. Great flirting is all about moving outside your comfort zone and finding your wow factor. This book will encourage you to be an edgier version of yourself – without going too far. We've all witnessed the ferocity of real life flirts and potty-mouth look-at-me ladies. They're out there, languishing in pubs, clubs and bars – putting on show-stopping performances, with head turning results. They're the ones hogging all the beer goggle attention. For all the wrong reasons. Which is fine if that's what you want. But being a tart is not what this is about. This is about saying, `what the bollocks!', developing some attitude, flexing the flirting muscle and going for it.

Let's start by establishing some facts about flirting. It can be intensely sexual but it's not just about sex. Flirting is about popularity, social networks and personal confidence. There are two types of flirting. There's flirting for fun and social advancement which is what we'll be doing right from the word "go". And for the more experienced flirts amongst us, there's flirting with intent, where you heat things up with a view to getting a date or, much, much more! A word of warning though, flirting with intent must always be practiced with caution. Only go there if you're prepared to go "all the way". Flirt Divas aren't prick teasers – end of story.

So what makes a Flirt Diva? Is it the art of the bump and grind; the ability to execute a 360-degree nipple tassel manoeuvre or the gumption to hurtle and hair-flick around the room and be a walking, talking, sex bomb?

*This Flirt Diva thinks not.*

The Flirt Diva is bold and sassy. She's the naughty fun one of the group. One part cheeky and two parts cocky, she has a real can-do attitude and a zest for life. She's all about sharing the love, channelling the good vibes and making an electrifying connection and an unforgettable impression. She's outgoing and funny and expresses herself through hi-energy day-to-day communication – not the sleazy stuff. She knows how to laugh at herself and act like a lunatic. She'll always wink and smile, and stop for a while to road test her cheeky banter. Her flirting superpowers extend beyond looking pretty and acting like a dim-wit. Like all great Flirt Divas, she knows that beauty comes in second to personality and brains in this 21$^{st}$ Century Flirt-Off.

Contrary to popular belief, the best flirts are neither the prettiest nor the most anorexic amongst us. In fact, more often than not, the great beauties don't have a clue how to exercise their flirt muscle because they've never needed to! They've spent a lifetime depending on their looks to get

19

by. So always remember, beauty does not thy best flirt make. The real qualities are get-up-and-go, dynamism, independence and a lust for life!

Good news for those of us who simply don't have the luxury of supermodel looks, or *natural* flirtability. It means we've got no choice but to be sassier and smarter to keep the banter bubbling along. That's what makes a killer flirt – women with sexual confidence, healthy self-esteem and strong identities. Women who know the subtle difference between aggression and assertiveness, sexuality and sensuality.

### *Don't-Ya-Wish-Your-Girlfriend-Was-Hot-Like-Me?*

There have always been flirts. Foxy, ditzy, insatiable flirts; kittenish, sluttish, subtle flirts and shag-me-happy-flirts. These Jedi Master Flirts have been frolicking, flaunting and out-foxing their competition with attention seeking wizardry right back from the days of the traditional Geisha girls.

For these girls, flirting is a way of life. Blessed with the most expressive eyebrows since Garbo, the best flirts *create a need* rather than satisfying it. They make an impact wherever they go in a world where their charm becomes an addiction – rapturous applause will do that to a girl. Getting a great response wherever she goes keeps the Flirt Diva happy and ensures her ego is always topped up, to the verge of bubbling over. Even when it's not, there's enough in reserve to keep her chugging along. She's the little Flirt Diva who could!

The art of flirting and body language is vital when it comes to understanding and interacting with the opposite sex. Perhaps you've toyed with the idea, but never quite got the hang of how it can be a direct hotline to success and romance. But that's the beauty of flirting. It's ninety percent instinct and inner confidence. Knowing that you're living life to the full, making an effort with your presentation and communicating effectively.

And while it's not just about dripping sex appeal, the super flirt is more than capable of morphing into a show-stopping sex object whenever she puts her mind to it. *"Don't read anything into this,"* she says as she leans over and kisses him on the neck. These ladies know all there is to know about creating a blistering sense of intimacy. That's what makes them hot. Great flirts never try too hard, it just comes naturally – after lots of practice that is!

The most positive way to get the vibes out there is through mind boggling, body frazzling practice, practice and more practice. The best flirts do it in their sleep and they do it with anyone or anything – man, woman, animal or child. So long as it's got a pulse, they'll flirt with it. These are the ladies that inspire and excite, that's why we're drawn to them. You can see it in their smiles and feel the love beam from their eyes. They're genuinely shiny, happy people who are all the more impressive because of the confidence they ooze. They're the ones we want to be around.

Make it your business to flirt with anyone and everyone, from your barman, barista or bookshop seller, as part of your training. Sure, you might find it a tad strange at first, but once you get cracking and start perfecting the Flirt Diva Commandments, you will begin to feel comfortable about putting it out there. You'll be flaunting your flirting tools like a pro in no time at all.

Flirting is both verbal and non-verbal. It's not what you say, but *how you say it.* It's all about the body language, not just the signals that you throw out there, but the ability to *read and understand the body language used by* others. It's a particular way of *being,* that tells someone you enjoy their company very much.

First impressions are based on your facial expression and your body language. How do you carry yourself? How do you come across at first glance? Are you smiling or scowling? Hunched over or standing up straight? What expression does your face fall back to when you're driving, reading, shopping or relaxing? Go and have a look in the mirror. Give yourself a "first impression" rating out of 5. And take a tip from master rapper and Mr Beyoncé, Jay Z: *"Smile into the mirror, you'll get smiles back. Throw insults into the mirror, you'll get insults back."*

Once you appreciate that body language is king, and you get the knack of reading it, it's a hell of a lot easier to suss out whether your flirt-mate has any clue at all about this flirting malarkey, and most importantly, whether he's playing the game.

Make no mistake flirting is a Point and Click tool that will help when it comes to navigating your way through these tough and ruthless times where the anything-goes romantic rules are relentless.

But don't get the wrong idea, this is not meant to turn you into an oversexed nympho, and it's not a ten minute wham-bam-flirting-slam guaranteed to get the man! This is about learning to recognise the positive signals as they come hurtling towards you, while also clocking the flirting signal failures – and breakdowns. Most of all it's about feeling comfortable in your own skin. Flirting keeps us young. Imagine how good you'll look with that fresh rush of lusty energy. Look at Madonna, still flirting like a goddamn madwoman!

And don't worry, it's not all selfless. Don't ever underestimate how the lethal combination of charm and cheekiness can make you feel. It can top-up your ego when it's running lower than low, and pep up your step. It can exhilarate beyond belief and give you that extra oomph to get up and jump right back in the ring, ready for another round on what might otherwise be the longest, lousiest day of the decade.

There's also scientific evidence that flirting keeps you glowing with a PMA – Positive Mental Attitude. The more you flirt, the better you feel and that's a good thing, not only for you, but everyone around you. The endorphin rush that you get from flirting is similar to the happiness hit you get when you bite down on a bar of chocolate. What further evidence do you need that flirting is the hottest way to stay healthy – physically and mentally? Try one-a-day and see how much better you feel!

Now that you're feeling feisty and all fired up for action, let's start the proceedings with a signed declaration to take this love therapy seriously. Make this your pledge to follow the plan, and declare your intention to be the most loved up you can be.

If you genuinely want to move forward in the relationship stakes, it's simple – just work with me here. Stop faffing, Banish those mental gremlins and think saucy little minx. Fill in the pledge below and start flirting!

*Let's hit it Flirt Divas...*

MY GET-LOVED-UP-ACTION-PLAN

**I, [insert name]………………………………………….**

**Agree to take the Get-Loved-Up-Action-Plan**
**I will complete the Fill-out-And-Keep-Flirt-A-Day-Tasks**
**To the best of my Flirt Diva ability**
**With a view to giving my lifestyle a complete overhaul**
**And thereby graduate with a**
**School of Flirt Therapy**
**<u>Flirt Diva PhD!</u>**

**Signed……………………………………….**

*All hail the Flirt Diva, she who will be Queen*

**Dated from …....….............and to…………………..**

*Witnessed by Sue Ostler, aka Flirt Diva*

# Step 1 Psycharazzi: How to psyche up like a Flirt Diva

*Week 1*

This week initiates your psycho-sexual recovery. The tasks, challenges and exercises are formulated to get your adrenalin pumping and shake your central nervous system. Expect to feel challenged, confronted, nervous, apprehensive, sad and excited all at once. The end result will give you the clarity of mind to broaden your boundaries whilst you prepare to explore new flirt-zones with less fear and baggage.

**Key phrase:** *Psycho-sexual self-survival.*

**Challenge:** *Confront those demons head-on.*

**Goal:** *Detox your mind.*

**Result:** *Lose the fear and flirt your head off!*

## Chapter 1. From Victim or Vixen

OK, we've established that your goals are to be bold and sassy, have a fabulous life and maybe even get zapped with an explosion of romance. Great! You've come to the right place to make that happen. So, we're going to pull out all the psychological stops and put you in the spotlight while we talk about flirting in terms of what *you* want to get out of it, and just as importantly, what *you* have to offer in the relationship stakes.

The focus right here and right now is *you*. You're special and you've got your own brand of flirtiness and quirkiness – so let's get it out there on the table. In case you hadn't realized it, you've got what it takes to meet, a good, no a *great* partner, and be part of a healthy, happy relationship. That's a very special skill to have, but it can always do with some zhushing up.

Step 1 of the Get Loved Up-plan is devised to get your flirting mojo rising by figuring out how you really feel about all this luv-stuff, whilst opening up your mind to endless new possibilities. It's all too easy to underestimate the value of the Single Phase, yet by focusing on self-improvement and developing as an individual, you're free to pursue all your own interests without any compromise. Yes ladies, this is a once in a lifetime opportunity when it comes to:

- Allowing special friendships to flourish
- Generating a hectic social life and a guilt-free existence
- Learning to create confidence within, rather than depending on others
- Being completely and utterly spontaneous

At the end of the day your inner flirt can always do with a top-up. Give yourself a break. Get ready to do something that's good for *you*. Something nourishing and enlightening. Move onwards and upwards and reconnect with the world again.  Don't do it for me. Do it for yourself!

This is all about acknowledging the need for change. Clearing the emotional slate, finding snappy new ways to get back into the romantic zone and learning to ooze confidence – do you remember how that feels?

Almost everyone has had a visit from the self-sabotage monster at some point. So let's deal with those feelings now to ensure you don't get an unwelcome visit later, *when it does count*. For example when you're out feeling hot, hot, hot and Mr Omigod! turns up – and you've got no idea what to say or do!

The shock of dysfunctional relationships or romantic malfunctions can leave us reeling, as well as savaging our self-esteem. Perhaps you've been through the washer when it comes those brutally ego damaging relationships? If so the aftermath can leave you all bruised and bloody. And unless you address the way you're feeling and face up to facts, you won't progress, at least not in a healthy, meaningful way.

Think of the following as a great big multi-confidence pill, designed to zap those personality disorder bugs and avoidance tactics, and get you off that déjà vu merry-go-round. It's time to stop spinning around and making the same old mistakes.

In no time at all, you will be unearthing your *real* feelings concerning love, lust and all that jazz. Emotionally, it's all about understanding who you are; the space you're in; the space you'd *like* to be in and the kind of relationship you see yourself in. From that point, it's about managing your romantic expectations.

### *What you'll get out of your new flirting super powers*

As you work through the 6-week program, you will find mini-challenges which encourage you to think in terms of goals and the romantic direction you're headed in. Unblock your emotional tract for once and for all and experience what it's like to be a fully rounded person, or in this case – drumroll please – the great Flirt Diva!

Once you've acknowledged where you're at, or realised that yes, you are challenged in this area, you can start working on resolutions. But first you have to think about what you want and more importantly *why you want it.*

You will start by taking small steps as you work through the book and fire up a love plan about where you'd like to be romantically in six weeks, six months – six years! You will need to consider the choices you make as well. It's a chance to stop, take a breath and put your romantic views into perspective to get some idea of the bigger picture. This is about figuring out what you want, and what's good for you right now. Will it be Mr Right for Tonight, or the big Happy Ever After? Ask yourself whether your "target range" is limited, or bordering on completely unrealistic. And be ruthless – if your self-esteem is so low that you'd bag any Bob, Bill or Ben who beer goggles his way into your bed – it probably needs a good hard look at.

Whatever your state of mind at this point, there's nothing like a series of shock resistant procedures to get things underway. Over the next few chapters, we'll introduce a few new tactics to use in your day-to-day which will help bolster your confidence and allow you to road-test your newly developed flirt muscle as you step out onto the field.

It's time to ditch the denial, dread and all those dodgy downers that keep you from living to your full potential, and start to surge forward with your life. Over time you will take control of your flirting biorhythms. You might not see the results for the first couple of weeks, but by the time you've finished with this survival guide, you will have killed off that split personality which has seen you yo-yoing between extremes of self-confidence and crippling insecurity. Those bad boys won't be stalking you for much longer. Lust and Personality are your new middle names, *got that?*

The way you approach this love plan will affect your confidence, your popularity and prowess. You'll be out there practicing and preparing in the knowledge that – if you plan for it, it will come! And there's no excuse not to, since flirting's free and you can do it anywhere!

Once you get started it will be the most natural thing in the world to flirt with everyone you meet. You'll be busy planning and scheming, always on the look-out for fab new flirt-ortunities. It will be bye-bye Anxious Diva and Hello Self-Assured Diva. You'll be a captivating gung-ho social butterfly with a calendar chock full of events, dates, parties and who knows, maybe even a hot new man in tow.

### Wah! Why can't it be more romantic?

Of course like anything worthwhile, it will take some effort, but if you don't put in the time, it will be all too easy to get distracted, with the end result that certain areas of your life will remain badly neglected. If you've come out of a long relationship – it might be your friends. If you're overwhelmed by your career – it might be your love life. Lord knows it can be tricky trying to juggle everything but if you've let the romance thing slide, or put it in the Too Hard basket because there's been too much going on, it's time to refocus.

Exciting? Not necessarily.

Essential? Absolutely!

Bottom line, don't be afraid to get your hands dirty for the sake of the L word!

Flirting your way to the top of the A-list is really no different to tending to relationship maintenance. The most successful relationships require time, work and TLC. We don't throw our hands up in the air when the relationship starts to fizzle and decide not to fix it because – that's not romantic!" Likewise, who in their right mind wouldn't want to be clued up about finding Mr Right? The best things in life *do* require effort.

I hate to state the bleeding obvious, but you *do* need to be clever, and you *do* need to use your nouse and your noggin. Not in a manipulative way, but in the same way you use your smarts and resources to get ahead at work or at college – in a thoughtful, purposeful way. Even if you've been in this flirting game for years and you think you're at the top of your game, it's not enough. Not in today's competitive climate. That doesn't mean bitching or bull-shitting – it's exactly the opposite. It just means you'll be a little better today than you were yesterday, and you'll try a little harder. That's what gives the Flirt Diva the unfair advantage.

Likewise, you need to have some idea of your *market value*. Because realistically, how can you sell yourself to somebody fabulous if you don't know your own value. I'm sorry if it doesn't sound very Mills & Boon like – but tough! As well as being a hopeless romantic, I'm nothing if not a pragmatist. So if you're thinking about stamping your feet and groaning and whining about why you have to make so much effort – I'll tell you what – get over it! Times have changed. We need to change with them. It's an open and shut case.

The moral of the story is – it does require more effort and chutzpah, but you *can* have your cake and eat it too. You just have to strap on your big girl brain and think laterally. Likewise you need to be prepared to take a risk here and there. It's that simple. And deep down I think you know that. You've picked up this book so you're clearly ready to move on. You're hankering to make some progress and honey, that's exactly what we're going to do. Consider this your formal man-ucation, the knowledge is all here. And stop stressing – it's a well known fact that Boy Wonder *always* shows up the minute we stop searching.

Now we'll crank through the action plan and work together to build your foundations, develop your check-list and decide on the deal-breakers as we start to unveil your flirt-onality.

*"I didn't blossom until after college. I think that was a blessing. It made me depend on my personality and humour instead of my looks."*
- Eva Longoria, Hollywood poster girl

## *Chapter 2. Revamp your emotional life*

This is the part of the Get-Loved-Up-Therapy which details your romantic history and monitors where you're at. You'll be surprised how much clearer things become once you write them down. It becomes easier to spot recurring mistakes and destructive habits – always useful when it comes to avoiding them like the plague next time!

Get ready to confront your right brain/left brain demons, as we tackle the Big Issues. Yes, the very ones that are sabotaging your lofty flirt ideals. It's time for a massive personality overhaul. *Take it all the way Team Flirt.* Nothing says "I'm over you loser" like a hot makeover.

Likewise, you will need to consider the origins of your flirting style (or lack of) right back from your formative years. The way you present yourself, your femininity, your social confidence, your personal style – even your career choices. It's crucial that we consider all this background material when it comes to understanding your psychosexual profile. This is what kick-started the development of your Flirt Backbone and supports the woman you've blossomed into today – it's powerful stuff.

So what are you waiting for? It's time to release some feel good emotional energy and breathe again. Open your psyche to endless new possibilities as you work through your mental to-do list. Go forth and embrace the challenges and hit them head-on. Once you accept that your symptoms are part of a bigger problem, you can focus on giving them the attention they need, and in doing so, *you will get on top of them.* If it's a serious issue and you need counselling, then please, book yourself in and come back to base when you're ready. Otherwise, keep reading, and prepare to make some big changes. Your cocktail, shaken not stirred reinvention starts here.

Get the ball rolling by opening up the 'love-vault' and thinking about your romantic history. Start by prompting your mum, your brothers and sisters or friends for clues about the way you approached the freaky puberty phase and beyond. Reminiscence about the men in your life. Try to remember how you felt about yourself as a teenager, the way you connected with boys, your brother, your father, your mates. Who were your idols and the rock gods you worshipped: the pin-up boys, pop princes and hormone inducing love idols? What do they say about your taste today?

Describe the impact they had when it came all things love, lust and libido. When did you first acknowledge aspects about your flirting persona that you liked? Or realise that what you were doing was effective - or not? What were the patterns that repeated themselves? How would you describe your flirt-onality? Were you an extrovert or an introvert? A natural flirt or a man-eater? Shy or gullible? Or were you so painfully awkward that nothing much ever happened? What were your weaknesses? Did your insecurities come through loud and clear? Did your nerves stop you from Going There?

Think about your personality with all its idiosyncrasies and quirks. Whatever you think about your qualities, there isn't anyone else on the planet with your DNA. You're an original through and through and we're going to hone in on your differences. Celebrate them, don't hide them!

The key to unlocking your inner flirt is seeing how all the different bits and bobs from your past are linked to form the style of flirt you are today. This will be your all-access pass to Flirt Divadom. Knowledge is power and power is survival. Just ask any super flirt, they're the ones that feel good in their own skin.

As you reconstruct your romantic history, you'll be in a rock solid position to retrace your flirting footprint from the very first moment it emerged. These are the crucial clues that will give you the know-how to live and love like a Flirt Diva. So keep thinking about your experiences and once you get to the challenges at the end of the section, write them down in your Flirt Diary, and when you do, be honest.

But don't expect this emotional roller coaster ride to happen without a fight. The idea of sitting down to sort out your issues and confront your personal demons *can* seem overwhelming. That's why we're going to rewire your brain first, and make a plan devoted solely to you.  This is about your body, your health, your emotional well being. The crucial thing is to reach out and really take the time and trouble to address the issues head on, and allow the survival instinct to kick in *before you hit rock bottom.*

### I remember my lowest time

Who doesn't? It was way back after The Break-Up. I was wallowing around in self-pity, too down on myself to do or feel anything. I was lost, confused – a complete zombie. I needed to get out of my own head, reinvigorate my life, and sort myself out. I needed validation. I wasn't looking for it from anyone else though. I had to find it within. And I had to start afresh. I didn't have any choice. I couldn't have sunk any lower. The shock hit after I moved cities in a bid to lick my wounds and hopefully recover. I woke up one sunny morning and it dawned on me that I didn't have a single friend in the new place, which, in the big smoke of a massive city made things a zillion times worse. I should have seen that identity crisis coming a mile off. But sure enough, the minute I made a commitment to sit down and confront my demons was the beginning of the long, slow climb up a silver lining.

Likewise, you can think of this as your chance to finally get on top of your weaknesses. Whether it's CSS – Chronic Shyness Syndrome, or a simple case of always chasing the wrong guys. And stop talking yourself out

35

of it! Kill those lust-busters for once and for all. It's easy to say "No!" but so much more satisfying to say "Go!"

It's the same when you disentangle yourself from a bad relationship, or dump that sorry sad-sack of a guy that's been keeping you down for too long. It's about taking a risk. What is the name of that fantastic book by Susan Jeffers? *Feel the Fear and Do it Anyway?* Uh-huh. That's what I'm talking about! Likewise when it comes to thinking about the kind of man you'd like to be with – do you really see the whole picture? Or are you focusing with your narrow lens. Only stopping to look twice if McDreamy fulfils your impossibly long checklist. This is not about lowering your standards – simply about *widening* your options. There's a whole world of opportunities out there, but you'll only see them if you take your blinkers off.

Think of it this way – of course you have high expectations about your romantic life, we all do – but rather than thinking in terms of what *he's* got to bring to the table, why not think in practical and psychological terms about what *you've* got to offer missy? Because it's all very well being oh-so choosy when it comes to picking a mate, strolling through your mile long Must-Have! lists, narrowing the margins and making it seemingly impossible for any man to fit in to your OTT expectations, but frankly, what does he get out of it?

What do you have that good old McDreamy can't resist? I'm not talking about superficial stuff, like your hot bod or gorgeous head of hair, I'm talking about the Real Stuff. The qualities and characteristics that separate you from the pack. What makes you so perfect? Are you in all honesty the emotionally developed super human that you'd like to be? How does your romantic history stack up? Have you been guilty of overpowering somebody, smothering them or pushing them away? What mistakes have

36

you made? Do you even know where you went wrong? Do you have a clue? And what makes you such good girlfriend material anyway?

I'm sorry if I seem brutal but these questions and more are pertinent when it comes to even *contemplating* a new relationship. Because I'm sorry, it's not enough to just sit around being pretty and witty, you've got to have the emotional maturity to deal with a relationship and all the madness that goes with the territory. The whole Getting Over It and Getting On With It process is a total Catch 22. And no matter what, you'll never beat it when your self-esteem is at an all time low. The only way of combating it, literally, is to jolt yourself out of your misery. We all know how hard that can be, but blessed is the Flirt Diva who is ready to move on and do whatever it takes to put the spring back in her step.

## When self-pity becomes your methadone

Let him go - if he was the one, he wouldn't be making you feel like this right now!

## Step-1
### Fill-Out-And-Keep 7-Day Flirt-Sheet

*Day 1.* Opening your Flirt Diary.

*Day 2.* Completing your Romantic CV.

*Day 3.* Recruiting your Flirt-Squad.

*Day 4.* Killing the Self-Sabotage Gremlins.

*Day 5.* Ditching the baggage and clearing the slate.

*Day 6.* Working on your Personality Profile and your FAB's.

*Day 7.* Scrolling through relationship choices and 'types'.

### Operation take-charge

1.  Clear the decks.
2.  Open your Flirt-Diary (preferably a blank A6 notebook).
3.  Write the heading: Step 1 – Emotional Admin.
4.  Turn the phone off!
5.  Close your eyes and clear all *negativity* from your mind.

# DAY 1
## STARTING YOUR FLIRT DIVA DIARY

Get the ball rolling with your Flirt Diary which will enable you to track your progress as you kick-start your flirtastic new life. Think of it as a tool which you will use from this point onwards to develop your Flirt Profile.

### Setting up your goal-keeping sheet

During this study of "you", it's important to pay special attention to what you want in both in the long and short term. Sometimes the only way to achieve this is to write down a wish-list of your hopes and dreams and goals. I use this system and update it every few months to keep myself on track. I call it my Dream-Chart.

*An example the areas of focus to get you on your way:*

Overcoming obstacles and stumbling blocks

Topping up your self-confidence levels

Setting relationship goals

*The activators could be:*

Get rid of things that are holding you back

The chance to start afresh

*The resources you will use:*

Personal experiences

Input from family, friends and Flirt-Squad (you'll find the details outlined on Day 3's Challenge)

**To get started you simply need to:**

- Mark a date in your diary for 6-weeks time.
- Write down everything you'd like to achieve between now and then.

*A note on Goal Tracking*: In order to stay on track, it's useful to keep your eye on the big prize. So think really hard about your most desired outcome. Is it to improve your overall confidence, come to terms with your past, or to get over your ex? Or is it to develop your sex appeal and get loved up?

**List your Top 5 goals**

*For example:*

*1.* Need to widen my social group

..............................................................

*2.* Learn new stuff

..............................................................................

*3.* Get out more!.........................................................................

*4.* Feel more confident....................................................................

*5.* Enjoy life more...........................................................................

*Write down what you need to do to improve*

*1.* ..................................................................................

*2.* ..............................................................................

*3.* ............................................................................

*4.* ..........................................................................

*5.* ........................................................................

**Remember:**

➤ Start with small goals i.e. getting out more, improving your fitness and broadening your friend network.

➤ Set realistic deadlines.

➤ Use the Flirt Diary to keep track of goals and monitor your progress.

*Now ask yourself where you like to be romantically in…?♥*

Six weeks ……………………………………………………..

Six months……………………………………………………

Six years……………………………………………………

## Happy-Snap: Believe it and it will happen technique

*Use the technique of elite sportspeople: Rebecca Adlington who won gold for Team GB in the Beijing Olympics has since said her motivation was, "this medal hanging around my neck." She could "feel' it." Apply it to your day-to-day: career, weight loss, bank balance and of course, relationships. Think of it as taking an internal snapshot of your new and improved flirt status. Simply start to imagine the person you want to be.*

*You want to be sociable, smart, sassy? So that's how you behave! By acting that way, you will begin to feel that way naturally. File the internal happy-snap away so that every time you're feeling low, or losing motivation, you can log on and call up a particular image to focus you. Whether that's finding a new partner or a new job – just visualize it and call that image into focus as many times per day as you can. Go easy though, it's addictive.*

---

♥ Think of this as opening your Flirt Account, it's dead easy to open and it comes with 24/7 flirting opportunities and access to romance worldwide. Apply online for more details of the Flirt-Diva Account today at www.vodkaandchocolate.com

# DAY 2
## MAKE A LOVE PLAN

*My name is:*

………………………………………

*My first kiss was with:*

……………………………………….

*My first boyfriend was:* ……………………………………….

*My first sexual encounter was:* ……………………………………………

*My great love was*: ……………………………………….

*My first break-up was:* ……………………………………….

*My fave boyfriend would describe me as:* …………………………

*My worst boyfriend would describe me as:* ……………………………

*My greatest romantic disaster was:* ……………………….

*List your last relationship/s including how long the partnership lasted and why it broke up:*

1.

2.

3.


*Now give yourself a score out of 10 for your level of happiness within each relationship*

1.

2.

3.

*Ask yourself whether you're ready to move on, or you're still grieving the loss of previous relationship/s. Tick:*

> *Yes*
>
> *No*

*In moving forward, can you describe your Mr. McDreamy? Tick:*

> *Yes*
>
> *No*

*Tick the reasons you'd like to be in a relationship in order of importance:*

1. To help bolster a flagging lifestyle
2. Looking for some thrills and spills
3. Because "all my friends are doing it"
4. To complete an already fulfilling life

Now list your Top 5 personal-to-do list. This is the stuff you want to conquer while *you're still single*. Best to figure it out now *before* you get hooked up!

*1.*

*2.*

*3.*

*4.*

*5.*

# DAY 3

## RECRUITING YOUR FLIRT SQUAD

OK, it's time to round up your Flirt Squad – a small group of mates who you'll invite along for the ride. Start thinking about who you'd like to invite to get the party started. There only needs to be one or two of them for this to be effective, but the more the merrier. Even better if you get a male member onboard as well, someone who won't be a dick about it, but will give you honest feedback from The Male Perspective.

The role of your Flirt Squad will be to push you, pull you and do whatever it takes to ensure you put your all into this. They will be required to support you unconditionally. If you are tempted to revert back to your bad habits (and less than flirtatious self), they will be there to pull you up by the bra-straps! In order for them to do that, they need to know that you're taking this seriously and *counting on them* as your support network.

The thinking behind the Flirt Squad is simple – flirts love fresh company to spark off each other, so you will thrive in the company of your wing-women. Not only will you have support on hand whenever you need it, but it will also make the forthcoming challenges more fun!

## Get your Flirt Squad cracking:

*1.* Make your Flirt Squad invite list.

*2.* Select a night for a Flirt Squad summit.

*3.* Turn it into a Girl's Night In with treats – prepare cocktails and cupcakes.

*4.* Welcome your recruits with celebratory drinks all round. Cheers!

*5.* Tell them about your pledge to carry out the Flirt Challenges over the next 6-weeks. Let them know that their encouragement is vital.

*6.* Explain there will be challenges that will involve them dressing up, checking out new places and having fun. Nothing too arduous!

*7.* Emphasise that they'll need to come with you on girl's nights from time to time *without* the boyfriend!

## Flirt Squad Rules

All members of Team Flirt are there to support *you*. That's the whole idea!

*Terms and conditions:*

- Your Flirt Squad has to genuinely love you enough to want to see you happy.

- They will ply you with feedback – and the occasional stiff drink.

## Flirt Squad Sing-along

*Flirt Divas Are Doing It For Themselves! (to the tune of Sisters Are Doin' It For Themselves – Eurhythmics.)*

*Flirt Divas are doin' it for themselves*

*Standin' on their own two feet*

*And flirting on their own!*

*Flirt Divas are doin' it for themselves*

*Thank you my lord, we did it ourselves!*

# DAY 4
## SELF SABOTAGE JUNKIES

Sometimes it is hard to acknowledge our bad habits and it can be impossible to stop, just like any addiction. These destructive forces can be both energy sources and energy zappers – powerful enough to send us reeling and prevent us from moving on. But sometimes the things that are addictive (and bad for us) can also be comforting to hold onto. It has a lot to do with what's going on under the surface. Any mail-order therapist will tell you that a great deal of what happened to us in the past, searches for expression in the present. Let me ask you this. *Have you dealt with your crap? Or swept it under the carpet?*

The only way to break through the self-destruct cycle effectively is to fight off the negative emotions which are at the core of the problem. If you're going through a phase where you're experiencing depression on one hand and loneliness on the other – it's not likely to go away until you *adjust your mindset*. This is *the* perfect time to confront the problems and address them head on. Hell hath no fury like a Flirt Diva scorned. Use that anger to motivate you into doing something positive. Get out of the zombie zone. Clear the fog. Get mad, get sad, and get pissed off. Express your emotions and let yourself *feel* the things of which you are afraid. Write down the worst thing that can happen, the worst thing that *has* happened. Look at the source of the emotion. Write down any "woe is me" stories in your Flirt Diary. And see how much more in control you feel once you put it `out there'. You've got to be really determined to let the bad stuff go. It only works if you're one hundred percent willing to stop being a victim.

When you've done that, ask yourself, honestly, what you need to do to get on top of the situation. Whether that means going gangbusters with the aid of this program, overcoming your issues with professional help, or getting a little help from a friend. Sometimes the solution can be as simple as taking a big breath and reaching out to trusted friends and family. But you do need to spell it out and tell them what you really need – they're not mind readers. If you need productive feedback – not just sympathy – shout it from the rooftops. There is no point walking around looking glum in the hope that others will somehow figure it out and hand you the magical cure. You've got to know what the problem is and know how to ask for help:

1. Write down what's triggering your sabotage tactics e.g. – fear of rejection.

   ----------------------------------------------------------------

2. Describe how life felt before – during a phase when you were in control.

   ----------------------------------------------------------------

3. List the lifestyle changes that need to happen in order for you to move forward.

   ----------------------------------------------------------------

4. Address the core of the destructive behaviour – *why are you feeling this way?*

   ----------------------------------------------------------------

5. What are the things that are upsetting you, draining you and stopping you from living the life you deserve?

-------------------------------------------------------------------------------

6. When have you felt this way before and what did you do then?

-------------------------------------------------------------------------------

7. What can you do to get yourself in a more positive state?

-------------------------------------------------------------------------------

8. Write down any recurring self-sabotage patterns.

-------------------------------------------------------------------------------

9. Now list solution driven ways to prevent them.

-------------------------------------------------------------------------------

## DAY 5
## *FROM VICTIM TO VIXEN!*

We've all had the emotional sucker punch, but if you're single and looking for a relationship, or just a good time, the first thing to do is get the hell out of emotional rehab. Often we're held back by fear and memories left over from our last relationship or traumatic experience and that's how we're left with baggage. So ask yourself this:

- ➢ Do you have big wads of emotional baggage?
- ➢ Are you prepared to check it in?
- ➢ Ready to dispose of it for once and for all?

Good, get packing! Often the baggage we cart around is the dregs which tell us that, regardless of how we might kid ourselves, we're not completely Over It. Or, if we do find ourselves in a new relationship, the Baggage Gremlins are likely to mess with it. So if you've battled problems and challenges (either as a kid or as an adult) and not yet dealt with them, it's likely they'll resurface as issues not yet resolved. For that reason, and for your own personal happiness, you need to bring a lifetime of baggage to the fore and get it out in the open. Only then will you be able to rid yourself of it.

You'll know instinctively when it's time to ditch whatever it is that's holding you back. It might be something abstract, such as memories or regrets from your last relationship. Or it might be something more tangible in the form of photos, mementos or emails. All the things that can haunt you and taunt you about the time you spent together. That's when it's time to devise a way to get rid of your baggage so you no longer feel trapped by it,

49

or by the temptation to lock yourself away and get all maudlin and messy after a few glasses of wine.

So if you're serious about cleansing yourself of the past, you'll need to be focused. And you'll need to tell your Flirt Squad beforehand. If you don't want them to mention Mr Old News! let them know! Then let the fun begin. A "goodbye ceremony" will give you the closure you need and help get rid of any baggage. It might be as simple as packing up the memories, the photos and locking them away, out of sight out of mind. Or it could be more elaborate and involve putting all the bits and bobs, emails and photos into a flameproof bowl and burning them (Kate Moss apparently did this after she broke up with Pete Doherty.)

Having looked at the past, identified patterns, and confronted the baggage, it's now time to clean the slate and get into a positive state with a closer look at You!


*And burials…*

After Ronnie Wood dramatically left Jo Wood for the teen Russian, Jo revealed to the Daily Mail how she 'buried' her wedding ring:

"A well-wisher sent me a coffin ring box out of the blue. When I opened it, I just thought, 'how fabulous!' I did a little ceremony and in the ring went."

# DAY 6
## PERSONALITY PROFILE

Before we can talk about relationships, the first step is to define yourself – who the hell are you? Who do you most aspire to be? There's a super woman in all of us just waiting to burst out. And while most of us have an idea of who *we'd like to be,* it can be a long trek across a shaky bridge that's keeping us from *where we want to be.* Your challenge is to get to the other side of that bridge where you'll be greeted with mountains of new found confidence and bling-bling attitude.

So let's have a look at how you're doing. How *is* your self-esteem these days? If you can't measure your self-esteem on the dipstick, you need to seriously work on topping it up with whatever attention it needs. In order to do that, you have to look within and honour your inner diva to really get on top of things. This is deep man!

## Cleanse your mindset

Get rid of the negatives and focus on every single positive in your life. Stop thinking about what you don't have and remind yourself of what *you do have.* In other words, the good stuff:

**1. Tick any of the following that apply to you and add in any other good stuff…**

**Currently I have a:**

a. Comfy flat

b. Generally good health

c. Decent job

d. Promising career prospects

e. Good network of friends and family

**2. Now write down 3 things you *love* about your life right now.**

    1.

    2.

    3.

**3.** What are your best qualities? Shortly I will ask you to make a wish-list with the qualities your perfect guy would have, but for the moment concentrate on how *you* shape up. For example if it's compulsory for your man to be fit and healthy, now's the time to check your own level of fitness and fabulousness!

So if you expect him to be

    *1.*   *Educated (and employed)*

    *2.*   *Outgoing and social*

    *3.*   *Honest and genuine*

    *4.*   *Fit and healthy*

    *5.*   *Image conscious and well groomed*

You might want to check how you match up in those areas. Give yourself a score out of 5 for each of the following:

1. Educated (and employed)
2. Outgoing and social
3. Honest and genuine
4. Fit and healthy
5. Image conscious and well groomed

## 4. Reinforce your positives: (and ask your Flirt Squad to contribute)

1. What are your relationship strengths? e.g Loyalty

-------------------------------------------------------------

2. What are you remembered for from previous relationships? e.g Honesty

-------------------------------------------------------------

3. What do you like most about yourself when you're in relationships? e.g Faithfulness

-------------------------------------------------------------

4.    **Now list 3 reasons that *you're* the best catch on the planet. Answer Yes or No if you are:**

1. Funny?
2. Good fun to be with?
3. Supportive?
4. Consistent
5. Considerate
6. Loyal
7. Tolerant
8. Compassionate
9. Sympathetic
10. Understanding

5.    **Now build your Top 5 most happening qualities into a really positive sentence about yourself. e.g *I am a healthy, red-blooded, fully functioning, sexy as hell woman!***

   ……………………………………………………

   ……………………………………………………

   ……………………………………………………

   …………………………………………………...

   …………………………………………………...

6.    **Find out what *you* have to offer in the relationship stakes.  Add Yes or No to the following:**

1. I have a strong relationship track record.
2. I've managed past relationships well.
3. I'm ready to move forward.
4. I'm free of my emotional baggage.
5. My emotional I.Q. is in excellent shape.
6. I'm so over my ex.
7. I understand the reasons the last relationship/s didn't work and I've learnt from it/them. Next!

*If you answered "yes" to more than four of the above, you're ready to move forward.*

*If you answered "no" to more than four, you've got more "inward" looking work to do.*

**In which case you need to go back over Step 1, highlight your areas of concern and start writing down solutions that you can start working on now, before you go too much further.**

**Now fill out this profile to get some fresh insight into what makes you tick. Here's a sample to get you thinking…**

| Personality Profile |
|---|
| **1. I like myself most when…**I'm social and happy |
| **2. The thing that scares me most is…** losing my friends and family |
| **3. I know I can avoid anxiety attacks by…**being honest and open |
| **4. I feel most positive about myself when…**I'm productive and motivated |
| **5. I feel at my most negative when…**I shut myself away |
| **6. The people I enjoy the most are brimming with…**positivity and lust for life |
| **7. My strengths are…**determination, passion, loyalty |
| **8. My weaknesses are…**stubbornness, prone to depression, self-doubt |
| **9. My ambitions in life are…**to maintain happiness and equilibrium |
| **10. I hold myself back when…**I'm feeling defensive |

*Now you try it…..*

---

**Personality Profile**

1. I like myself most when…...…………………………………………………

2. The thing that scares me most is……………………………………………

3. I know I can avoid anxiety attacks by………………………………………...

4. I feel most positive about myself when………………………………......

5. I feel at my most negative when…..………………………………………….

6. The people I enjoy the most are brimming with…..……………………….

7. My strengths are…..…………………………………………………………

8. My weaknesses are…..………………………………………………………

9. My ambitions in life are…..…………………………………………………

10. I hold myself back when…..………………………………………………

---

**<u>Bring on the confidence boosters!</u>**

Now think back to a time when you felt your best; when you felt the closest to super woman that you've ever felt! And before you say you can't remember such a time, there is sure to be some photo or some memory that will trigger this day, this phase, this feeling. So think hard! You've been there before so can get back there. The trick is in planning the steps you need to take to recreate that feeling and what strategies you need to unleash.

**1. List the top 3 things you hope to rid yourself of over the next 6-weeks**

1. Negativity about the break-up – can't let it go
2. Shutting myself off from friends
3. Wishing I could be someone/anyone else!

*Now you try*

1.

2.

3.

**2. Which of the following do you need to do in order to feel strong again?**

- Get closure from previous relationship/s
- Work on getting my confidence back
- Acknowledge that I am ready to move forward with my life

*Now add in your own:*

    *1.*

    *2.*

    *3.*

**3. In order to progress, you need to know who you are – and what you've got to offer. Give yourself a tick for each of your strong features:**

1.     Smile

2.     Intelligence

3.     Sex appeal

4.     Good listener

5.     Cheeky

6.     Warm

7.     Non-judgemental

8.     Witty

9.     Easy to talk to

10.    Funny

11.    Silly

12.    Approachable

13.    Mischievous

14.    Down to earth

15.    Authentic

**4. Make a list of every compliment you've ever had. Rummage around as far back as you can to come up with every single nice thing anyone's ever said about you!**

1.

2.

3.


## Market value or FABs – Features and Benefits

OK, so we all agree that it's a tough old battle zone out there in the world of romance, and in order to be on the front line, you really need to think about your FABs: Features and Benefits. What are they? Describe in 25 words what makes you different – thrillingly so? How can you showcase your FABs if you don't know what they are?

**Finish this sentence:**

What makes me so unique is and gives me the potential to be the Queen of Fabulousness is:

...............................................................................................................

...............................................................................................................

...............................................................................................................

**How do you feel about every aspect of your life right now? Give yourself a score out of 5 for each the following. And be honest!**

Looks

Personality

Dress sense

Beauty maintenance

Fitness levels

Health

Employment potential

Skills/accomplishments

Commitment to friends and family

**Now add up your total score.** Total:

If it comes to less than 20, you've got some serious work to do girlfriend! That means breaking it down into bite size bits and focusing on your weakest areas.


## Victim or Vixen? Fear and how to conquer it.

*It's never easy, but it can be easier – if you reinforce the positives:*

1. You've got to believe in yourself before you can convince anyone else to believe in you.

2. Remind yourself about your FABs on a daily basis.

# DAY 7
## RELATIONSHIP CHOICES AND "TYPES"

Assuming that a relationship is on your goal list, it's time to put some thought into narrowing it down to the *right kind* of relationship. Let's get you out of your comfort zone and into trying something new. That means stepping outside your romantic "type". Ditch the saying: "He's not my type". Haven't you ever walked into a shop and tried on a dress that "wasn't your style" only to find that it sucked in your waist, enhanced your breasts and somehow, fantastically, elongated your legs? It happens. Mixing and matching "types" was an ongoing theme for the *Sex And The City* girls. They knew they had to date outside their "type" in order to find the prince and they got involved with all sorts of men that we didn't expect – neither did they. They went outside their comfort zones and in the process they learnt to appreciate that there was more to men than their wallets, career prospects and sex appeal!

The only way you'll ever really know what works is by experimenting, which is simply one more process of educating yourself about romantic opportunities. It just might open up something completely different and wonderful than what you'd expected. You'll never know unless you try.

*"He was like the flesh and blood equivalent of a DKNY dress – you know it's not your style, but it's right there, so you try it on anyway."*
- Carrie Bradshaw.

### *What's your type?*

Think of those women who seem so perfectly suited to their partners, you know them, those "perfect couples" whose marriages suddenly break-up. Because, newsflash, they were never really happy, *they just looked good together.* Something to think about if you're committed to trying only one "type". It might be the worst type in the world for you, but you'll never know because you won't experience any other "types!"

*Is your thinking about what you will and won't accept is too limited?*

What's your "type"?

Must he be tall dark and handsome? Write it down whatever it is.

...................................................................................

*Now cross it out!*

Make a promise that you will no longer be limited by the narrow restrictions you've placed on yourself.

*"I don't have a type. It took me this long to narrow it down to gender"*
-Ellen DeGeneres (US chat show hostess married to actress Portia de Rossi)

### 1. Write down you wish-list:

It's fine to think about what you want – so long as it doesn't focus solely on the shallow, superficial stuff. This is about finding a well balanced, healthy relationship of minds - not just builder's biceps!

Is it realistic to expect Johnny Depp's looks, Simon Cowell's bank balance, Brad Pitt's fathering skills and David Beckham's physique? Not really, no! You've got to be honest with yourself. Think about the kind of person you're likely to attract and the qualities that are most important to *you*. Not your mates, not your mum – *but you!* Remember to think broadly. He could look perfect on paper but be as dull as dishwater in real life.

**Your checklist should include the fundamentals. For example:**
*Wanted: Emotionally intelligent man, who isn't freaked out by the "R" word (r...r...r...esponsibility).*

## 2. Confirm your deal-breakers

Stick to your guidelines when it comes to the Big Issues: beliefs, values, moral code and religion (if that's important to you). This is not about the colour of his hair or his height. It's the big things that are the real deal-breakers. Think of them as your non-negotiables. For example:

- You will not compromise on sexual preference – he really cannot be gay!
- Nor should he be a repeat sex offender.
- Or a serial rageaholic.

**Write down your Top 5 Deal breakers (in other words, he must have):**

*1. Ethics*

*2. Honesty*

*3. Emotional I.Q.*

*4. GSOH*

*5. Responsibility*

**Must he be compatible with your:**

- ✓ Race/religion
- ✓ Values
- ✓ Age range

**List the qualities you're attracted to in the order of your priorities.**

**My list looks something like this:**

1. Honest
2. Genuine
3. Smart
4. Sensitive
5. In touch with his feminine side
6. Good Sense Of Humour
7. Outgoing/fun (can bring something to the table)
8. Emotionally available
9. Educated (hopefully)
10. Employed (hopefully)

*Now list yours:*

1.
2.
3.
4.
5.
6.
7.

8.

9.

10.


***Putting it altogether:***

- Accept that moving on may be hard at first and that your new life will need a helping hand.
- Concentrate on getting your "inner-self" back in shape.
- Quit the blame game – negative energy doesn't help!
- Tighten up your ethics radar – two wrongs don't make a right.
- Hard-wire your new PMA (Positive Mental Attitude) into your DNA.


OK!  Time to chillax and take a breather. The most effort you need to make now is to come up with a "seasonal resolution" that just means a resolution for any season.

What's yours? Think about it now and decide which 3 specific things you'd like to change the most.


1.

2.

3.

***Flirt Alert:*** Make a pledge not to be trapped within the confines of your rules.

- 1. What are the rules that govern your love life?

- 2. Write them down………………...............................

- 3. And now ladies, step away from the rules!

*"My list is all about balance. You can have smart but not funny. You can have funny but not very smart. You can have intellectual but not social. But I want it all!"* *"I don't do anything half-a\*\*ed and I want someone who can keep up with all that."*
- Cameron Diaz

### *Flirt Review: Finding your Signature Flirt Profile*

It's time to fill out your Flirt Review. You will do this every week at the completion of the step you've just worked through. This is an essential part of the process of discovering your 'romantic self' and eventually revealing your signature flirting style.

The Flirt Review is not meant to show anyone else, it's simply a private way for you to get your feelings out. The idea is that it allows you to track your flirting journey, look back over the highs and the lows, and identify the areas you need to work on. By mulling over your approach to every aspect of your life, you will start to see a more vivid picture emerge, and eventually your individual style will be revealed.

Approach it in the same way you would a normal diary and allow yourself a good fifteen minutes to respond. Under the Flirt Review heading write down any thoughts that come to mind about this process of confronting the past. Consider the following as you jot down your thoughts:

1. How has the emotional self-work affected you?
2. What areas do you need to keep working on?
3. What is the main goal you will work towards as you leave behind the negative parts of your old life?

You can comment on the bigger picture things as well – dreams, disappointments – your dissatisfaction with the world! Who knows, down the track you may be in a position share your wisdom with others who need it – your sister or cousin, or even further along – your daughter!

# Congratulations you've completed your Step 1 missions!

## Step 1 Learning Outcomes
### Key Points

> ➤ Successful flirts are comfortable in their own skin.

> ➤ Find out who you are – and celebrate that person.

> ➤ Get rid of your FAD (Flirt Anxiety Disorder).

### Checklist

✓ Self Knowledge

✓ Courage

✓ The desire to move on

**Vamp Mantra:** *This is not a quick fix. It's long term!*

# Step 2 Flirtarazzi:
# How to vamp up like a
# Flirt Diva

*Week 2*

In Step 2 we'll get cracking on the A-Listers and find out what makes them such damn good flirts! It's time to live and breathe the essence of the women you admire. What do they have and how can you get it? Get ready to swot up on your favourite superheroes as you go through the next seven-day challenges.

**Key phrase:** *Pro celebrity flirts.*

**Challenge:** *Research your idols and study their tricks and tips.*

**Goal:** *Let your role models and superheroes inspire you.*

**Result:** *Find your celeb match flirt style.*

### *Chapter 3. From Geishas to Garbo to Girls Aloud*

So what have we established so far? That there's more to flirting than hair-raising-head-flips and shag-me-senseless smiles. Correct! Flirting is an attitude – a way of life. It's not just a ploy to lure the fellas – you can flirt everyday to your heart's content. It's a living, breathing buffet of power moves designed to give *you* the social advantage. And that's what we'll be concentrating on here. The following chapters will open up your flirt vein and get you thinking about who your favourite flirts are and why.

Now that you've had a good look inwards, it's time to think about how you want to tweak, improve or re-position your outward persona. Whether you want to be a bigger, better more assertive version of yourself, or develop a more subtle approach, there is without a doubt, a naughty flirt out there in celeb land with a particular style that you can relate to, or aspire to. FYI, for me, it is all about those women with a heady concoction of flamboyance, sophistication and rock 'n' roll pizzazz.

Yes but can they flirt? Well I hope so, it's part of the job description! And since there's no escaping them, why not make the most of them? Don't hate them for their looks and notoriety; learn instead from their talents.

In a culture obsessed with youth, sex and image, flirting is the new black, but it's always been there, lurking in the shadowy background. When I look back at the super divas from a bygone era, I shake my head at their mind-blowing powers of seduction. They've got it all over us 21$^{st}$ century gals. Let's go back in time for a brief overview at the history of the worlds' greatest flirts before we fast forward to our contemporary role models.

Hands up who knows any real-life heavy duty flirts? I mean the fire-breathing temptresses who gobble up men for lunch – the man-eaters! You know them – the killer heels, masses of lashes and more cleavage than seems humanly possible. I'm not just talking about the girls from the post-

Jordan age of exhibitionism, or the Madonna brand of strapping, sexualised superwoman – I'm talking about the ladies from the golden age of Hollywood.

## So what makes a super diva: Attitude? Ambition? Drive? Energy?

Once upon a time flirting was an art form performed with theatrical aplomb. The olden day flirt may have been regarded as coy and enticing, but my, my, wasn't she also a tease, a gold-digger, a siren, a vamp and a vixen all rolled into one. Flirting wasn't portrayed as light-hearted banter back then, but to prowl, pick up, proposition and tease. In other words, flirtation was not a playful little ego boost, rather a means to a specific end. Straight from the school of *"when I'm good I'm very good. When I'm bad I'm better."*

Perhaps you've seen them in action, projected up on the silver screen where they've been immortalised in *film noir* classics. The great seductresses, sexually ruthless and unwaveringly feminine; elusive, and captivating with an air of simmering mystique. Who were those white hot goddesses?

Mae West – queen of the one-liners. Marlene Dietrich – mistress of the micro-expressions, a tiny barely perceptible facial movement which left men staggering. Greta Garbo – a sex bomb who left audiences gasping with a well timed wicked flash of her brow. The unshakeable charms of Lauren Bacall, Eva Gardner, Sophia Loren, Vivien Leigh, Bridget Bardot, Liz Taylor – the list is long and it goes on. Picture Audrey Hepburn reclining on the pavement outside *Tiffany & Co*, her hair high-piled sky hair, those glasses, pearls and little black dresses. The when-in-doubt-pout unforgettable charms of Marilyn Monroe.

This brand of femme fatales led us to believe that flirting was about manipulation and sexual power. Nowadays that's just an antiquated notion. When it's done for the wrong reasons – to manipulate or play games – it's a setback for women worldwide, and that is *so* not what this is about. The femme fatale is just one old fashioned stereotype of the flirt. Today when we think of flirts we think of smiley, shiny fun girls. Right at this moment, Cheryl Cole is probably Britain's favourite flirt.

But it's not just images on the silver screen – we see the ghostly shades of the Hollywood goddesses imprinted on our modern icons – although their particular brand of sexuality has been watered down dramatically. Contemporary flirting has none of the art and more of the tart – a situation we hope to rectify here! The glamour and mystery has been somewhat passed over in the rough and tumble of the disposable pash 'n' dash culture in which we live.

As such we are very rarely encouraged to think seriously about this crazy little thing called charm. It's always about being skinny this and designer handbag that!

Flirting can never ever be too serious either, that's the point. Nor is it about showy display like in the days of old. On the contrary it should be effortless, seamless. It's just not flirting unless it's done with a twinkle in your eye and cupcakes full of banter. The same goes for seduction which we'll talk about it in more detail in Step 6. But it's not just about sex-appeal – it's having the Wow Factor.

What's the most memorable thing about a burlesque dance performance? It's not the bump and grind, but the *presence* of the dancer – the sensuality, the drama and of course, her charisma. It's just like sex symbol Sophia Loren said, *"Sex appeal is fifty percent what you've got and fifty percent what people think you've got."*

The best flirts are women who know how to put on their best face, showcase their strongest assets, flaunt their personalities and work their body language. That means being *aware* of the way they're coming across and the signals they're silently communicating. These are the ladies who know how to smooth talk their way in and out of anything. *You know them –* they charm their way out of tight spots, and away from parking cops. This Flirt Diva has talked her way out of being drunk, dumped and dismissed. Am I proud of it? Hell yeah. I just owned it. And so can you.

Do *you* know how good it feels to charm your way out of any situation? I'm not just talking about exploiting your feminine charms, I'm talking about using your smarts and thinking on your feet.

There's a whole world of mating and dating flirt rituals playing out in the public arena, and it's infectious seeing them in action. By now you should be starting to visualise how flirting can become a crucial part of *your* lifestyle. That's how the flirting pros do it – they have their own inbuilt flirt radars just like the one you're developing now. They don't reserve flirting just for romance or special occasions – hell no! They're prepared to go on the charm offensive at the drop of a hat.

*"His eyes have made love to me all night"*
- Greta Garbo, *Camille,* drawing her leading man to her with the simple and
expert delivery of one arched brow.

### *Chapter 4. Learning from the F\*\*\* Ups of the Flirt Divas*

Over the next few chapters, we'll study the good, the bad and the ugly of the celebrity pros and all the flirting styles in order to hit upon the one you identify most closely with. We'll channel your superheroes in order to activate your Vamp Mantra and find out what your signature flirt style is: hard 'n' fast, sweet and girly, mysterious, charming or – man-eater!

Before we do our crash course in CWS (Celebrity Worship Syndrome) and glide down the red carpet, let's put the spotlight on two very different kinds of Flirt Divas. First there are the Flirt Divas in making – that's you babe! You're the one who's been caught up in the hustle and bustle of the singles' scene for a while. You've been lurking and a hiding, beeping and a smiling, but now you're ready to leap out of the closet – resplendent in your sequinned playsuit.

Then there are the super divas. The queen bees of the pop hive, the babes of Britain, wild women of Hollywood and Celebrity Flirtstars. And ladies, they do have a thing or two to teach us. And why not? There's a reason these women are in the public eye – they've got something special to offer.

To begin with they're mostly performers of some sort or another (which is exactly what flirting is) so it makes sense that putting on the old razzle-dazzle, posing, pouting and posturing for the masses comes ever so naturally to them. Flashing those big crocodile smiles and making every one fall in love with them is as easy as walking the Chihuahua. That's their shtick. That's what helps them rake in the big bucks. They're as tightly coiled as snake-charmers and highly trained as Geishas when it comes to the art of flirting. Thanks to a privileged lifestyle which gives them all-areas-access to make them the super-ladies they are today.

In order to see how the fancy moves of the super divas can inject some va va voom into our own personal style, we need to narrow our focus down to the women we admire most. Appoint yourself "body language expert" and start looking out for the signals. Far more than just passing time, watching these gals in action is actually useful. This is no guilty pleasure, this is important business! That means the next time you're flicking through a magazine, pay attention.

### Celebrity Flirtstars: The Good, the Bad and the Ugly

Once upon a time when I worked for a glossy music mag, I spent every free night rocking in the front row of the best live shows on the planet. Holidays were spent jetting between the world's hottest music spots. Ten years on and my how I miss it. The outrageous VIP music showcases where I crammed in as many shows as I could, from glam rock to glum rock and queens of slut rock! All those amazing women, so little time: Blondie, Courtney Love, Madonna, Beyoncé, Gwen Stefani, Pink, Janet Jackson, Tori Amos, Alanis Morrisette, Sinead O'Connor, Marianne Faithful, Chrissie Hynde – Cher for God's sake! Oh *man,* that was the life.

My super heroines have always been a lifeline to my dreams and in many ways my true inspiration, the stuff that's fuelled my fantasies ever since my mum chaperoned me to see leather clad rock goddess Suzi Quatro – my first ever live rock concert and Omigod, I'd never seen anything like her in my life!

This formed the basis of my shiny, sparkly rock star fantasies. The superstars gave me hope. They represented freedom and showed me that I could be whatever I wanted to be. What incredible qualities did they have, and how could I get them? I wanted to strut like that, and do that crazy, sexy, cool thang. I wanted to flirt and charm and drip sex appeal *like that.* I wanted to perform in front of an audience and have them eating out of the

77

palm of my hand. But most of all I wanted to be successful and in control of my destiny. I wanted to do my own thing; to live and breathe the essence of the women that I admired and adored.

From that moment, I was happy to borrow techniques from the stage and screen queens and learn from them. I saturated myself in a sea of women dynamos – pretty much anyone with the balls to put themselves out there and do something! Having that focus got me thinking about what gave these girls their stardust, and more importantly, how I could get some. I wouldn't rest until I understood what defined these mistresses of seduction, and simply through studying them, I would. Thanks for the insight ladies!

So now it's over to you aspiring Flirt Divas, do you want to be a super divafied powerhouse up on a pedestal one day? To be at the top of your tree and as successful as can be? To be treasured by your clients, colleagues, friends and lovers? I know I do! So I'll look to the experts for tips on how to get there. And that's what you're going to do as you get into the heads and minds of the women you admire and adapt bits and bobs of their best qualities.

Which super Flirt Divas do you most identify with? Who are your icons, goddesses and inspirational heroes? Is she a sports-star, movie star, political tsar, lobbyist, teacher, actress, singer, burlesque dancer or stand-up comedian? Has she won an Oscar or a Grammy or been nominated for public office? Has she done something, anything amazing lately?

We will study our idols in exactly the same way these ladies studied theirs. Madonna has confessed to being equally inspired by the German movie goddess, Marlene Dietrich and the Mexican artist Frida Kahlo; while Kylie Minogue has revealed her "girl crush" on bisexual 20s screen icon Tallulah Bankhead made her want to "release her inner Tallulah."

Think of the women that have become a significant part of your life thanks to their high profiles; tough, sexy women in control. The only way to nail down their mysterious, seductive qualities is to study them. You will find at some point, just when you need it, that a succession of images begins to flood your brain; images from the stage and screen: flirts living, loving, lusting and excelling.

You will get a chance to write down your list of your superheroes at the end of Step 2, but start thinking now. And remember, this is an age-free zone – just look at women like Helen Mirren, Joanna Lumley and Sophia Loren who show us it's cool to be hot, gorgeous bikini babes even in your 60's!

And what's this got to do with flirting? Only everything. It's a reminder that we do have to be sexually savvier and more open-minded when it comes to our romantic lives. They do need to be tweaked and tightened to fit within the new guidelines; monitored and scrutinized in the same way that our careers and friendships are. It's just plain lazy leaving it to chance. Especially if you have goals that include motherhood and marriage! You can't be taking that stuff for granted. I don't care how old you are! In this day and age it does need thought and planning – if you want a long lasting partnership that is. We *do* need to do be all over things to ensure we've got matters in hand. And if a closer analysis of the super divas can help in our pursuit of a fabulous life, then bring it on; we'll take anything we can get!

But ladies, if there's one thing I have learned, it's that whatever else you think about these mega-stars, you must never look to them to take the lead in your quest for finding long lasting love. In this area they are quite simply not the experts. *Erm, did someone say Jen Aniston?*

Let's face it, the super divas are not exactly winning any Grammys in the healthy relationships categories. They may be mega talented when it

79

comes to looking good, but that doesn't help in the game of love. And when they have a hard time of it, boy do we know about it.

They go public with their scratch-your-eyes-out custody battles, dodgy adoptions, cheating husbands, and seductive nannies. They get cheated on and dumped just like the rest of us, only ten times worse because the glare of the spotlight is upon them. Well you tell me how Posh felt when David was doing the dirty with that Loos woman and it made front-page news around the world? Or how Sienna felt when Jude shagged the nanny? The point is, just because they're the richest, the thinnest or the blondest – it doesn't mean they get the boy! Even Kate Moss had the bitter taste of betrayal and humiliation as she was publicly two-timed with a younger and possibly more beautiful model during the Pete Doherty phase. Gasp!

But since they're the ones in the limelight, they're the ones leading the pack. And keep in mind, these artfully mussed super chicks didn't ask to be idols. Or as put so succinctly by soul diva Ms Amy Winehouse, *"I'm not in this to be a fucking role model."*

But for the moment at least, they're stuck with it. So are we. And since the role models we choose influence our approach to life, not only in love and sex, but all things image and dating related, it's hard not to get sucked as their lusty lives and red-hot sexy liaisons are played out for our voyeuristic pleasure.

We're not here to talk about their relationship skills (or lack of them). Nor should we try to emulate their SDR, Severely Dysfunctional Relationship style. But it is useful to study their flirting styles to get some insight about how the A-Listers drip, drip, drip charisma. There's a goldmine of stardust to be mined here courtesy of the masters which you'll start to identify with. And whether you love them or hate them, it's all food for thought designed to get your head into the flirt-zone.

Just one more thing before we get started. There is a notion that if your self-esteem is not as healthy as it could be, you should possibly ignore celebrity culture because it can make you feel even worse when you don't match up. Here at Flirt Diva HQ we say bollocks to that! Celebrity culture is very much alive and well and it's impossible to ignore. So rather than trying to avoid it, why not exploit it and take the positives from it? So long as we remember it's OK to be inspired by the super divas, but it's not OK to get too carried away with it!

So clad in my Burberry trench coat and Jackie O glasses, I set off undercover to study the signature flirt styles of the celebrity divas. I've made my selection based on the world's most popular celebrities. My quest? To identify what makes them so gosh darn appealing. Now I'm sharing it all with you. So go and pour yourself a glass of something chilled and gather back here for the Flirt Divas are Doing it for Themselves discussion group where we identify the five main flirting styles.

## _Hard and Fast Flirts_

First up on the super Flirt Diva celebrity roulette wheel brings us the Hard and Fast flirts – starring no other than Madonna! Love her or loathe her, you can't leave the world's most successful artist out of a conversation devoted to flirting powerhouses. She is the ultimate. Her theory clearly being, if you've got it, flaunt it!

Madonna has been rocking the slutty queen of pop thing – forever. Through her music, video clips, films, sex books and any other medium she can get her hands on. What's her secret? Courage? Steroids? The ability to take risks? To believe in herself with death defying conviction? To not give a flying fuck what other people say?

Who remembers the film _In Bed with Madonna?_ The stakes were high, the cameras were rolling and the movie was set to become a world wide blockbuster. But the High Priestess of Raunch still took that gamble and ran the risk. Did you see the way she flirted her heart out with Latino heart-throb Antonio Banderas? Regardless of the fact that he was there with his wife – who looked not only foxy, but fiery as all hell.

The point is that Madonna – hailed as one of the most influential feminists of her time – isn't afraid to put her yogified arse on the line. You can say what you like, but she's got balls, and thanks to her "I've always been comfortable with my masculine side" attitude, she's not afraid to admit it. Not long before they divorced, she confessed that ex-hubby Guy Ritchie had encouraged her to "hone her feminine side" Perhaps he didn't realise it's not really in her DNA!

> _"I'll flirt with anyone from garbage men to grandmothers."_
> -Madonna

## _Mysterious Flirts_

Then there are the Mysterious Flirts. Who will come up when we roll that wheel? Why it's – Angelina Jolie! Firstly she's obnoxiously beautiful, _and_ she manages to pull off her Mother Teresa role with aplomb. Just look at her bewitching transformation from hell raiser to Saint Ange quicker than poor old Jen could say, "you're having _another_ baby!?" Compare the "now and then" photos. It's not just the pearls and twin sets that sit snugly in place of the skin-tight leather that's made us think differently. It's her body language, her posture and the way she holds herself. Take a look next time you see her photographed. It's noble and so very regal. From bisexual bombshell to Global Ambassador of the world. How quickly we forget the fury we felt when La Jolie brazenly reached out and lured a then married Brad Pitt right into her sticky little honey-pot.

Study her "camera face" and you'll see that she's got two or three classic poses down pat. There's that soft, gentle, maternal smile where love just beams right out of her eyes. Then there's the man-eating grin, and of course, The Sultry Look. Angelina's secret weapon when it comes to flirting is to keep us thinking of her as Aphrodite – the ultimate sexual goddess. As evidenced by her comments during her last pregnancy when she cooed. _"It's great for the sex life. It just makes you a lot more creative. So you have fun, and as a woman you're just so round and full."_ Hmmm.

## *Sweet Girly Flirts*

Sarah Jessica Parker's, Carrie Bradshaw, is the classic sweet, goofy girly flirt. And while she may not have conventional good looks, it's all about her style – and it nets her gazillions. Added to that she has a quirky, vulnerable quality which makes us warm to her all the more. Cameron Diaz is another. A self-confessed "boy crazy" actress who admits to *still* breaking out into pimples at the sight of a hot boy (and this in her 30's). And yes, she does have a Diaz-tastic body and a killer smile, but so do loads of Hollywood actors – the difference is that she's all about being a goofball! And she'll happily say so in every interview she does. She's got a warped sense of humour and she's a big kidder. That sense of fun comes through on the big screen and we respond to it. So it's not just men that flock to her, women love her as well.

## *Charming flirt*

But do you know who I've always had a soft spot for? She is the definitive charmer. It's Hollywood's former wild child Drew Barrymore, not so much because of her looks, in fact if you study her closely you'll see that she's not a classic beauty at all, certainly not in the league of some her peers, but Drew has something else, something that both men and women find completely irresistible. It's called Charm and it's flirting's big sister.

Drew's got this whole flower-child-hippy-thing going on which is all the more intriguing because, she's also one of the most successful women in Hollywood. And it's not only her acting – she has her own production company and was one of the top-dog producers in the multi-million dollar, box-office hit *Charlie's Angels.*

Remember this is a woman who clocked up the rehab miles from the tender age of 14, but went on to become a freaking powerhouse. While she's as smart as a whip, incredibly hard-working, ambitious and successful, there's something about her that's soft and vulnerable.

Her twin personalities Super Flirt Diva Vs Woman Child are rolled into one luscious package designed to make her less threatening than many of her peers. She doesn't come across as one of those Hollywood dames who start throwing diva strops once they obtain a level of success. She gets there on her wits and intelligence but *still* manages to come across as just a wee bit ditzy, and *always* up for a good time. Somehow she's managed to hold onto something precious from her childhood. There's a twinkle in her eye and a smile that says, "I'm fun. Why doncha' come on over and see for yourself". Yet, you can be sure that once she puts on her serious hat, the gloves come off and that business brain whirrs around at dizzying speed Grrrr!

## *Mischievous Flirts*

Then there's your Mischievous Flirts. winner of the 2009 Woman of the Year *G.Q* Award, Ms Lily Allen, defines this one – she's a natural. Whether she's off her face and acting like a tit, or just being cheeky. I mean look, anyone's boob can pop out of their extremely low cut white t-shirt on the one day of the year they've forgotten to wear a bra, but twice in one day? Naughty Miss Allen!

If you saw her in action on her short lived TV chat show, she was all giggles, naughty smirks and fluttering lashes. It may not have worked for TV ratings but you could see the boys she interviewed were falling for it big time! Lily's a super flirt and she knows it. So much so that she's even happy to reveal her trade secrets publicly. "*I start off being mates, I hit them in the arm and then it's only a matter of time before I've got their penis in my hand."* Yikes! Is this what Cheryl Cole was thinking of when asked what she thought of Lily Allen and she replied, "Chick with a dick."

*"Well behaved women never made history."*
- Christina Aguilera

*"I used to flirt with girls just to get the guys circling around us. I'm getting out of it now. I have to look after my reputation."*
- Katie Price (*before* she divorced Pete).

## *Step-2*

### *7-Day-Fill-Out-and-Keep-Flirt-Plan*

**Day 1.** *Breakfast at Tiffany's.*

**Day 2.** The Super Divas in action.

**Day 3**. Who's your favourite flirt and why?

**Day 4.** Chick Flick Night.

**Day 5.** Babe with a Book.

**Day 6.** Body language Expert.

**Day 7.** Cooking up your Flirt Diva Profile.

# DAY 1
## BREAKFAST AT TIFFANY'S DAY

Round up the gals and plan a *Breakfast at Tiffany's* themed day. It's just an excuse for a fun, girly thing to do together. The good news is, that really can be anything at all, so long as it's got that element of glam to propel your Celebrity Pro Flirt mission forward.

If you decide to host at home, start by getting creative with the invite. Use a super glam image from the movie – a large hat and sunglasses should do the trick with the words "You're invited to party like Holly Golightly, dahling!" Have all sorts of fun finger foods at the ready, mini cupcakes and cucumber sandwiches, and ask your guests to bring Audrey-esque accessories: tiaras, long black gloves, cigarette holder, pearl necklace, fake lashes. Combine all the accessories, try them all on and mix and match a few different looks. Then style yourselves: lashings of mascara and hair up into the classic Audrey 'upsweep'.

Once you're all looking the part, watch the movie and if you're feeling really organised, host a quiz based on the movie. If practicality allows, take a road trip or a scenic train trip. You don't have to go far. Wear headscarves and over-sized sunnies. Pack a picnic and of course, loads of chilled champagne. Otherwise, plan brunch, afternoon tea, twilight cocktails or a garden party. Anything you can come up with to put you in the right frame of mind to for your forthcoming Flirt Diva world domination

## *DAY 2*
## *WATCH THE SUPER FLIRT DIVAS IN ACTION*

Think all-singing-all-dancing-Flirt-Diva and pick a live gig – it can be music, comedy, dance or theatre – whatever your preference. If it's music, step out on your own rock-chick tour by reconnecting with the tunes that make your world go round.  Or get out of the mosh pit and try the experience of a boutique festival – so much more refined dahling! Whatever you do, just make it your business to see as many live gigs as you can. Or if you're feeling really brave, register to audition for a talent comp. If there are no gigs accessible to you, have a DIY concert of your own. Gather up your gal-pals for a night of frank and-filthy girl talk, fancy drinks and vodka-soaked laughs – like a lingerie tonic for the liver. Watch the super ladies in action and think about how to interpret their killer moves. Host a danceathon, a bopathon, or a Madonna-thon. Crank up the tunes and psyche yourself up.

Spin a few discs and sing-along with your favourite super divas. Rock out your video-game console for some *Guitar Hero* or *Rock Band* fun where you can form your own entire band. Crank it out with karaoke, Singstar, Wi or a good old fashioned hairbrush! Re-enact those crazy teen rockstar fantasies. Listen to your voice, control it, lower it, sex it up. If you've really got a taste for it, record your own CD (though you will need to go into a sound studio to do this properly). Once you've done that, it's time to perfect the moves.

Leave your "cooler than thou" image behind and relive your teenage years. Practise your pose, preen and pout. Be completely OTT in a bid to engage your inner vamp and get in the mood. There's just no room for inhibitions here. This is best done over many, many glasses of wine with the very simple intention of having a laugh. The message is simple. Sexy comes from within. Babe magnets take risks, they know how to live in the moment, work a mic and shimmy on the dance floor. And if you don't believe that this stuff can work, listen to what soul diva Estelle has to say about it:

*"I was so star struck by Mary J. Blige, I just lost my mind. I hugged her three times, told her I loved her, and cried. I've loved her since I was 13. I learnt to sing to her. I didn't have vocal lessons; I just watched a lot of videos and listened to Mary.* - Estelle

## DAY 3
## WHO'S YOUR FAVOURITE FLIRT AND WHY?

Get the gang over and ask them bring their ideas about ladies who flirt. Start with a definitive list of all your leading ladies. Then ask the tough questions: who in your opinion is a good flirt and why? What do you love or loathe about them? What qualities inspire you? And finally, if you were a super diva, who would you be? FYI, my list would be a combination of all my favourites – and there are zillions!

And remember, they don't have to be famous to be on your list, so be sure to include your lesser-known super heroes as well. These days I actually prefer championing the underdog and supporting the artists and performers that we *don't* read about in the glossies – those with smaller profiles and cult followings. But don't get me wrong, I still love nothing more than an evening with Madonna or Beyoncé at the Wembley Arena or the O2 Stadium!

**Here are some examples from Flirt Diva HQ to get you thinking:**

1. Madonna – for being Madonna!

   *Signature flirt – Hard and Fast: in your face sexuality*

2. Lily Allen – a foxy, foxy girl

   *Signature flirt – Cheeky: brash in yer face cockiness*

3. Naomi Campbell – a real wild child

   *Signature flirt – Tough Love: sultry, tempestuous diva*

4. Gwen Stefani

   *Signature flirt – Sweet Girl: smiley and quirky*

5.  Shakira

*Signature flirt – Mysterious:  natural, unstyled and sexy as hell*

**Thinking as broadly as you can, write down who you rate as the best flirts**

*1...............................................................................*

*2...........................................................................*

*3...........................................................................*

*4.............................................................................*

*5.........................................................................*

**Now, just for fun, who do you rate as the worst flirts?**

*Example:*

Victoria Beckham? (Lose the pout love)

Jordan? (Stop telling us all your dirty little secrets!)

*1...............................................................................*

*2...........................................................................*

*3...........................................................................*

*4.............................................................................*

*5.........................................................................*

**Who do you rate as the most flirtable men?**

Simon Cowell: because he can make us famous?

Russell Brand: because he's an outrageous flirt and just doesn't care?

George Clooney: because he's timeless, classic – and swoon inducing?

## DAY 4

## CHICK FLICK NIGHT

Now for a Flirt Diva guide to flirting just like they do in the movies. Organise your Flirt Squad to hotfoot it over for a chick-flick fest and theme it chronologically. When I wanted to share the chick flick love, I turned the whole exercise into a Girls Night Out and shared my guilty pleasures around (this Flirt Diva is nothing if not generous). Start with the femmes from the Hollywood Age spanning the 40s/50s and 60s, before moving onto the 70s/80s/90s and finish with the contemporary Flirt Divas. As well as the classics, it's also great to study the silent movies to see how crucial the body language was. Oh, and don't forget to study the fellas' as they kick out the moves with their leading ladies.

One of my favourite Hollywood legends is Lauren Bacall, a sultry siren who left men shivering in her wake. Who can forget the film *To Have and Have Not.* The lucky recipient was Humphrey Bogart – the love of her life. The famous line was, *"You know how to whistle don't you, Steve? You just put your lips together and blow"* which she carried off at the tender age of 19. Smouldering like nobody's business! What a cool cat! I locked myself away and read her autobiography as soon as I laid eyes on her, and it did not disappoint – the all consuming love of Bogie's life until he died in her arms and she moved on to Frank Sinatra. Now that's a love story!

*I've made these film recommendations based on my own findings:*
- Audrey Hepburn in *Breakfast at Tiffany's*
- Dietrich in *Blue Angel,* Garbo in *Camilla* and Hayworth in *Gilda*

- The entire back catalogue of *Sex And The City*
- Madonna in *Desperately Seeking Susan* and *Truth or Dare*
- Every Monroe classic including *How to Marry A Millionaire* – just to ogle the looks and poses!
- That husband stealing bee-atch, Angelina Jolie in *Mr and Mrs Smith*
- Beatrice Dalle in *Betty Blue*
- Jane Fonda in *Klute* – Electrifying.
- Kathleen Turner in *Body Heat*
- Linda Fiorentino in *The Last Seduction*
- Katherine Hepburn in *Holiday*
- Jennifer Beals in *Flashdance* – watch out for the infamous lobster eating scene. Slurp!
- A very young Drew Barrymore in *Poison Ivy*
- Sally Hawkins in *Happy Go Lucky*
- *All* the Hitchcock classics – famous for featuring the world's most notorious ice-queens

# DAY 5

## BE A BABE WITH A BOOK

Now that you've narrowed down your list of leading ladies and included anyone you've ever admired – it's time to read up! Many of your super divas will have published biographies. Depending on when it was printed, they may be hard to find, in which case you will need to source Amazon, your local libraries or beg, borrow or steal!

Right then, time to get reading! Devour everything you can to give you the full picture. Make this your bedtime reading.

*The biography list which instigated my Flirt Diva awakening:*
*Remarkable*

- Hilary Clinton – fascinating for the voyeur in us all.
- Elizabeth Taylor – the stuff of which true heroines are made.
- Nancy Reagan – bizarre!
- Kate Moss – the woman doesn't speak, so it was never going to be very revealing was it?
- Courtney Love – now there's a real life hellcat.
- Lauren Bacall – spellbinding.

*Revealing*

- Drew Barrymore at 13 – total shocker.
- Jane Fonda – fascinating.
- Marilyn Monroe – I wish only to know what happened to that woman on that fateful night.
- Kylie Minogue – ho hum.

***Revolting***

- Sharon Osbourne – disturbing!
- Katie Price – why does she want us to know all that!

*"I love romantic comedies. I love reading love stories in literature, in film and in music. The idea of love is got to be what gets us out of bed every day and gets us ready in bed at night, hopeful for the next morning if we're not experiencing love."*

> – Drew Barrymore

# DAY 6

## APPOINT YOURSELF 'BODY LANGUAGE EXPERT'

It's time to get up close and personal with the women that sell the most magazine covers. There's a reason for their massive popularity and as you study their images, you will soon see patterns in the way they demonstrate the good, the bad and the ugly of flirting styles. So surrender yourself to the allure of the glossies and start flicking!

Identify the reason that Celeb A is looking so hot right now while Celeb B is looking spectacularly bad. Look at her facial expression – what it is saying? What do her eyes radiate? What does her mouth say? Is her smile genuine? What does it tell you about her? How does she stand? What does she do with her hands, feet, legs? How does she tilt her head; angle her body; position her smile? The answers are all here in black and white. Take notes and scribble things down as you flick through.

Next, study the "hot couples" and see if you can pick the genuine couples from the fame-seeking couples. Look at the way Brangelina and other A-list couples pose with each other compared with more "normal" couples. What's the difference between the "real thing" and the A-list couple and can you spot it?

*PERSONALISED FLIRT PROFILE*

# FLIRT DIVA FUN AND GAMES

## Phase 1 Creating your Personal Profile

The quiz will identify the celebrity flirting style that your style most closely resembles. You will be assigned a "celebrity flirt profile" which you will refer back to once you reach Step 6. At that point you will discover your signature trademark.

*Top Five Flirt Diva styles:*

1.  *Sweet Girly flirt*
2.  *Cheeky flirt*
3.  *Mysterious flirt*
4.  *Hard and Fast flirt*
5.  *Tough Love flirt*

**1. It's Saturday night and your girlfriends are missing in action. Do you stay in or hit the town in the hope of picking up?**

a) I'd call up my gay bestie and head out to a fabulous bar where there'd be plenty of prospective guys.

b) Definitely hit the town! Why waste a Saturday night in? I don't need my girls with me to meet guys.

c) I'd organise to have dinner with one of my married friends. Maybe they could introduce me to someone?

d) I'd take advantage of the situation and use the free time to catch up on work.

e) I'm not comfortable going out by myself to meet guys, so I would probably just spend the night in front of the TV.

## 2. You're out on a girl's night when your spot a really cute guy checking you out. Do you flirt with him?

a) A little, I don't want to let the opportunity pass so I'll give him my number and organise to catch up another night.

b) Hell yeah! I love my girlfriends, but this guy is hot, hot, hot!

c) Of course! But I make it clear that I'm not leaving my friends.

d) No way, it's just the girls tonight.

e) No, I'm having too much fun with my friends.

## 3. Would you try a less conventional method of meeting guys like online dating or speed dating?

a) I can barely get my mobile phone to work, let alone set up internet dating.

b) I don't need to. I manage just fine meeting guys in person.

c) No, I'm an old fashioned kinda gal.

d) Yes, I've tried them, there's nothing wrong with giving it a go.

e) I'm looking into it – I could do with the help!

## 4. Are your friends mainly single or loved up?

a) They're a bit of a mix, although I see a lot more of my single friends.

b) Single I guess. I don't see that much of the ones that are in relationships or married.

c) Most of my friends are loved up. I find it's a great way to meet men through their partners.

d) They're mainly from work, so they tend to be typically married.

e) A lot of my friends are in relationships, only a couple are still single.

**5. Do you spread the word about looking for Mr Right, or keep quiet about it hoping that one day he'll just materialise out of thin air?**

a) I talk about it, but I find it's better to keep having a good time. He'll come along when the time is right.

b) Who's looking for Mr Right? Mr Right For Tonight will do for now!

c) I put it out there, but I don't want him to sniff my desperation!

d) I don't believe in fate, so I definitely spread the word.

e) I tend to sit back and wait for him to come to me.

**6. When was the last time you asked a guy out?**

a) I gave my number to a cute guy I met just last week.

b) I don't need to ask. I put out so many signals that they always ask me first!

c) Never! I'm not that forward. I *never* will be.

d) In the last few weeks. I'm straight to the point and I don't have time to mess around playing games.

e) I can't remember. I'm clueless when it comes to putting put out the right signals. Most of the guys I meet become friends.

**7. You're at a swanky bar with the girls when you spot a really cute guy across the room. What do you do?**

a) Flash him a sexy smile and peek seductively over at while I have a laugh with my girlfriends. Once I see him alone, I'll find a reason to wander by...

b) Eye-ball him until I get his attention, then strut over and introduce myself.

c) Make a tiny bit of eye contact, then wait for him to make the first move.

d) Wander over and strike up a witty conversation.

e) Move my posse closer to him, then wait for him to approach.

**8. What's your number one way to get attention?**

a) Guys usually find me cute, quirky and funny.

b) Just one? Honey I ooze sexual energy, guys can't resist.

c) My adorableness, my charm and sweet nature.

d) My intelligence, ambition and personality.

e) My ability to be friends with guys. I get inside their friendship circle before making my move.

**9. You're sitting at a bar splitting a bottle of Pinot with a girlfriend when a cute guy comes over and starts hitting on you. You ...**

a) Crack a joke and initiate some lightly flirtatious banter.

b) Launch into a full-on flirt fest and bring out some of my best you're-coming-to-bed-with-me material.

c) Smile politely and send him some subtle sexy vibes.

d) Roll my eyes. A guy this cocky can't really be serious.

e) Feel a bit awkward. I'd love to know how to turn on some of that come-hither charm.

**10. Sleeping with a guy on the first date is ...**

a) Not ideal but if it happens, it happens. Sometimes, if the chemistry is there, you just can't help it.

b) No big deal. How do you know if he's worth keeping if you don't test the equipment?

c) A big mistake! No guy will ever want to marry you if you put out on the first date.

d) Typical. Most guys only want to go out with you to get you into bed.

e) Something I just don't do. I'm only just starting to get to know a guy on the first date.

**OK! Let's see which celebrity flirt you most identify with, before going on to develop your very own signature style in Step 6.**

**1. Mostly A's:** *Cheeky Flirt*

*Your Sex and the City Match is:* Carrie

*Your A-List Match is:* Lily Allen, Cameron Diaz, Drew Barrymore, Kate Hudson, Jamelia, Estelle, Agyness, Kirsten Dunst, Alesha Dixon, Sarah Harding.

**2. Mostly B's:** *Hard and Fast flirt*

*Your Sex and the City match is:* Samantha

*Your A-List match is:* Lady Ga Ga Madonna, Christine Aguilera, Rihanna, Sharon Stone, Paris Hilton, Dannii Minogue, Katy Perry.

**3. Mostly C's:** *The sweet girly flirt*

*Your Sex and the City match is:* Charlotte

*Your A-List match is:* Cheryl Cole, Gwen Stefani, Kelly Brook, Duffy, Beyoncé, Jennifer Aniston, Terry Hatcher, Mischa Barton, Jennifer Hudson, Holly Willoughby.

**4. Mostly D's:** *Tough Love flirt:*

*Your Sex and the City match is:* Miranda

*A-list Match:* Katie Price, Naomi Campbell, Janice Dickinson, Heather Mills, Pink, Tina Turner, Grace Jones, Courtney Love, Cher, Joan Jett, Nicole Scherzinger, Lindsay Lohan, Katie Price, Angelina Jolie.

## 5. Mostly E's: Mysterious flirt

**Your A-list match is:** Shakira, Dita Von Teese, Kate Moss, Scarlet Johansen, Keira Knightley, Uma Thurman, Daisy Lowe, Sophie Ellis-Bexter, Penelope Cruz, Chloe Sevigny, Hilary Swank, Alexa Chung.

**Oscar winning Halle Berry was named sexiest woman alive by Esquire magazine in 2008. The New York Daily News quoted her, as saying.**

*"I don't know exactly what it means, but being 42 and having just had a baby I think I'll take it! "Sexiness isn't necessarily what is on the outside. Sexiness is a state of mind a comfortable state of being. It's about loving yourself in your most unlovable moments. Does being the sexiest woman alive imply that I know a thing or two about what's sexy and, possibly, sex itself? I'm not sure, but here's what I do know: I know I'm dammed well sexier now than I used to be. Let me make an argument here, not so much for me, or even for y age being sexy, but for what I've learned. I've picked up a little over the years. Sexy is not about wearing sexy clothes or shaking your booty until you damn near get hit dysphasia; it's about knowing that sexiness is a state of mind – a comfortable state of being. It's about loving yourself even in your most unlovable moments. I know a little bit about that. Sexiness is also knowing what's sexy to you. To me, spaghetti is sexy, especially if it's served off the tips of a man's fingers, I like that. And I think wine is sexy, just before sex. It relaxes me. I think lingerie is sexy, and I'll wear it sure. But truth is, I'm good-to-go in a tank-top and bare feet – although every woman should own at least one pair of good pumps. That's really the only wardrobe you need for sex: a tank top and pumps. Another thing I know damned well is that at 42 I am sexier now than I used to be."*

***Flirt Review: Finding your Signature Flirt Profile***

OK, now that you've identified your "celebrity match", you should be starting to get a feel for your *own* flirting style. Write down any thoughts that come to mind about the ways in which you can use your new knowledge to further develop your own style. Consider the following as you jot down your thoughts:

1. Who are your influences and what is their impact on you?
2. What have you learnt from studying your idols?
3. How has it sharpened your ideas about the woman you aspire to be?
4. Describe the woman you aspire to be. What are her main qualities? What makes her so attractive?
5. What are the raw qualities you have to start work with?

**Complete this sentence:**
*I have what it takes to be a killer flirt because………………..*

…………………………………………………………………………

………………………………………………………………………..

………………………………………………………………………..

………………………………………………………………………..

# Congratulations you've completed your Step 2 missions!

## Step 2 Learning Outcomes

*Key points*

- ➤ Learn from the Masters.
- ➤ Retain your own sense of identity, but let others inspire you.
- ➤ Award yourself superstar status!

*Checklist*

- ✓ Super Diva inspiration
- ✓ Flirt Diva perspiration
- ✓ Lashings of stardust!

*Vamp Mantra*: *I am the Queen of the Universe!*

# Step 3. Passionarazzi: How to be hotwired like a Flirt Diva

## Week 3

Step 3 is all about taking a pro-active approach. It's designed to get you out of the house and out of your comfort zone! You'll find yourself moving outside your boundaries and experiencing new territories. Your seven-day Action Diva challenges are devoted to snazzing up your lifestyle and jazzing up your social confidence. And remember, the more invitations you extend, the more you will get back!

**Key phrase**: *Social Confidence.*

**Challenge:** *Developed a thirst for action and adventure.*

**Goal**: *Improved quality of life.*

**Result:** *New experiences and action-zones.*

***Chapter 5. Finding your Wow-Spot***

Step 3 is all about thinking big. How do you think the truly great flirts get to be that way? Not by sitting around guzzling champagne and chocolates whilst watching countless reruns of *How to Marry a Millionaire* – one viewing is enough! They actually get out there and do it. They live their lives in terms of world grabbing headlines: *"Roll up, roll up to see the greatest flirt on earth."*

Likewise when it comes to revamping your lifestyle, you have to want to get out of your rut and make yourself an active part of the solution, rather than locking yourself down in a sluggish, rigid lifestyle. Use your time on this planet to give the performance of your life. Attack it with passion and gusto. A simple change in your social calendar can kamikaze you out of your everyday hum-drum and into a socially frenzied whirlwind, where you're up for trying anything and everything. So for those of you who dozed through your under-graduate How-to-Find-your-Wow-Factor classes – welcome to a place called life. People flock here when they want to have fun. Think of this change to your routine as a confidence and motivational all-in-one multi-booster to kick start your fantasy fulfilment.

So what do you say? Are you up for it? Ready to recharge your life and take some risks? Ready to say "what the bollocks" and stand out in the crowd? To put your "bright ideas cap" on and push your personality out. Are you seriously committed to this idea of wheeling in the wow factor, whooping up the next few weeks and creating a crazily exciting environment for yourself? If the answer is great big, gung-ho, YES! Then you are way overdue for this personality transplant which is all about being proactive, not reactive! It's time to stop worrying what everyone else is thinking, and stay on track with your own dreams and desires.

So now, in the interest of becoming Action Diva and morphing from blah to bombshell, you'll need to get cracking with your new life. We're talking lights, we're talking camera and we're talking action. But first, let me indulge with a story about my most revered real life flirt idol.

### Once upon a time…

There was this woman who could out-flirt anyone – yup, even me! She is one of those maddening women who have men salivating and flocking to her 24/7. She can have them wrapped around her little finger in no time at all. *Bam!* She's not blonde. She's not thin. She's just FUN.

Her eyes sparkle, her hair shines, she has the biggest smile in the room and she adheres to the Flirt-a-Day-plan like a religious nut. She's a social butterfly, a style cat and a flirt-ninja all rolled into one. She knows all about the latest movies, books, music – and footy scores. She writes letters to the editor of her local newspaper; she paints, draws and indulges in more y-chromosome-man-friendly activities than anyone else I know. She invites friends over for garden tea parties and serves Vodka Melon Frappes and Red Velvet Cupcakes with Raspberries. *Bitch.*

Those envious of her assume she takes uppers in her drinks – *how else could she be so buzzy?* But it's not that – she's got stuff going on. It radiates from every pore of her body. She's Action Girl with good old fashioned pep-up-and-go and that makes her as sexy as hell. She has this way of placing her hand on the small of your back, hanging onto your every word, and tossing out the saucy grins like there's no tomorrow. There's just one word for it – seductive. This woman has excelled in the art of the binge-flirting and she works it like nothing I've ever seen before. There's something energetic and empowering about her. The bottom line is chicks like this are cool. And the best thing is – you can be a little minx just like her.

Thanks to a lifetime of practice Flirt Divas around the globe are leaping out of bed with toe tingling energy, ready to mount the merry-go-round of life and feeling positive about the day ahead. They apply their wham-bam super brand to all elements of life. And so should you. When it comes to vamping up your flirt appeal and social magnetism, you've got to think in terms of jazzing up your life. That's where you'll find the power to attract, mesmerise, hypnotise and make people *worldwide* crave your company. And quite honestly, the only way you're going to get that kind of ammo, is by squeezing as much as you can into this crazy little thing we call life.

The fun begins with Operation Break Out. The first step is to smash free of your old life and the stale routines. Only when this is done can your new life begin to take shape. Once you free the demons that have been holding you back, you will ricochet to a place where the experiences of hurt, shock and setbacks will fade as they are nurtured and repaired by feel-good therapy. I'm living proof! The secret is in knowing when it's *time* to take action. Prop yourself up, say "enough is enough" and make that conscious decision to get out of your rut once and for all.

### How this Flirt Diva got loved up

I knew it was time to take action during my single phase when I found myself getting dizzy from going around in circles. Eventually I sat down and thought about what seemed to be the problem. Then I grabbed my diary and listed the issues that were plaguing me. Somehow, the simple action of writing it down helped motivate me to actually get off my butt and do something about it. It was a weird time but ultimately life-changing. Since this book is partly about sharing my experiences with you – I'm going to tell you about it.…

110

It was during the wilderness years. A long, hazy blur of groundhog days where I would wake up, drive to work, slog away, drive home, eat, drink and sleep, and do it all over again the next day, six days a week – seemingly forever! It finally got to the point where I was starting to feel uncomfortable in my own skin. I had that uneasy sense that if I didn't start widening my horizons, soon they were going to close in on me. The bad vibes even started coming out in my dreams. I remember waking up in a cold sweat one night because of the claustrophic sense that I was living in a cardboard box! That's when it became clear I needed to shake things up – and I knew just what to do (spend enough time wallowing in your own pity-party and you will come out of it eventually).

I was well overdue for a change of scenery – more to the point, I was desperate for it. I needed soul food! What to do? Where to start? I thought back to the things that had rocked my world as a kid. What had I done then that would reinvigorate me now? I needed to reconnect with the essence of me. It was the only way I could see myself shaking the blues and getting my old self back – because god knows I missed her.

Like so many other teen divas, I had always had a thing about horse-riding. I hadn't been near a horse for years but I needed to now. I sat down with a copy of the local paper, found what I was looking for and booked myself in for a day ride around the local park. And wow, I wasn't disappointed. It was every bit as incredible as I remembered.

And I didn't stop there. I also craved time spent by the ocean. Two weeks later I was cruising down the highway for a weekend of surf, sun and sea. Ripping gleefully through the waves and bouncing about like the world's most carefree eleven year-old made me feel like an invincible mermaid. Somehow the sheer exhilaration and familiarity of the experience (and the early nights spent re-reading Enid Blyton) was *the* best way of putting myself back in touch with who I was, and *what I was all about*. So yes, it was every bit as brilliant as I'd remembered. And a gut-churning reminder that momentarily acting like a kid can change your outlook in the most excellent way. Give it a try!

A few weeks later, I successfully requested a four-week study break from my full-time job. I'd always wanted to do a course in scriptwriting but had never got around to it. Now there was a summer course available that slotted in perfectly with my annual leave and gave me the perfect breather. I can't tell you how good it felt to get out of the nine-to-five grind and back into student mode. What a relief to slide out of the power suits and schlep around in jeans and sneakers feeling like king of the kids! Not to mention the much needed confidence boost it gave me. Once I'd finished the course, I even dared myself to write a TV script and submit it to a network. It was never developed, but hey it was fun trying and it's something I'll always have to look back on.

I rounded off my period of transition with a seaside holiday – with my parents in their caravan. Talk about the ultimate regression back to childhood! But I never could have predicted the incredible impact that holiday would have on me. I took long walks along the beach every day and swam, snorkelled and detoxed my way to hi-energy health. Along the way I flirted with the hot German barman in the tiny tent next door; celebrated the New Year; made a wish under the full moon and I must have drank some love potion because for the first time in years, I felt alive. I felt feminine. I felt sexy and I felt in control.

Getting buzzed up on new stuff motivated me to find more fresh inspiration – I'd take it anywhere I could get it. After the hols, I did a mini city-break with a girlfriend where we partied the weekend away and flirted our heads off at every opportunity. And it didn't stop there; I felt like the world was my oyster. I took in live shows, performances – especially bands since music made my world go around. Often I braved the gigs alone since many of my "coupled up" lame-arse friends didn't want to come – but I wasn't going to miss out. And within weeks, at one of these gigs, I locked eyes across a crowded room with the man who is now my fiancé. And *POW!* That was it.

In hindsight, it wasn't that surprising either. Sometimes the simple act of jumping out of your comfort zone and landing in a different environment forces you to take a fresh new look at things. All these mini changes in my life had the domino effect of forcing me to start thinking and acting in another way. A typical reaction when you're exposed to new people and exciting experiences. The changes may not seem like such a big deal in the first instance, but down the track you'll start developing a lust for life that simply wasn't there before.

So there you go, that's my story – and since it evolved over a period of 6-weeks and included each of the 6-steps you're studying here – it became the love plan you're now reading! And really, who at the outset would have thought a few lifestyle changes could make you so much more susceptible to meeting the right partner? Well it worked for me! So the trick, lovely ladies, is to reboot your psyche by reinventing yourself. The reinvention starts here.

### Call a girly summit

In order to surge forward with your fab new life, you need to leave behind the old – starting with the negatives. And let's face it who doesn't waste good energy on those all consuming bitch-o-ramas with our girlfriends? But if ever there was a reason to dump the pseudo friends and spend the balance of your time with real friends who love you – and wish

113

only the best for you – this is it! Make as much time as you can for your Flirt Squad – the women in your life who will not only help you hit your stride, but support you, encourage you and cheer you on while you branch out socially, professionally and of course, flirtatiously.

Perhaps that was the real key to success behind the *Sex and the City* phenomenon. Sure the shoes, the labels, the bars and the men were one thing – but tell me this – who wouldn't die to have friends like those girls? We may not have it as good as the Fab Four, but we can still have the time of our lives with our Flirt Squad. Get your friends onboard as you work through the each of the remaining steps.

This is your time to let yourself go crazy and experiment. Research what's going on, rally the troops and get everyone motivated. Keep reminding your Flirt Squad how much their enthusiasm and support means to you. And be persistent. Call a girly summit and bang them over the head with your plans to jazz up your life. It may take bribery and corruption – but nothing a wine drenched pizza night won't fix! And the tiny financial investment will be minuscule compared to what you get in return. So think long and hard about the gazillion and one things you could be doing to propel yourself out of couch-potato-land and picture your new life – all decked out in garden-party-frosted-cup-cakes-and-fluorescent-pink-lemonade – spiked with vodka of course!

And remember, these are not just methods designed to meet the man of your dreams – though god knows they'll help – they're designed first and foremost to get you out there – living the dream!

### Finding your Wow-Spot

Right then, the first step is to prepare. Believe it or not, spontaneity is sometimes best when planned! Make a note in your Flirt Diary to start reprogramming your life flirty-first thing tomorrow! This is the time to blast outside your boundaries and hurl yourself into whatever it is you thrive on, whether it's your career, studies, travel or just plain fun stuff. Anything you want to do, you should be doing now. Now is absolutely the time to reinvigorate your mindset and start going for it. This is YOUR TIME. Because right here, right now, you're calling the shots. You can do what you want, when you want, with who you want – you're a free agent. But, always remember – your current status is temporary. You've got the opportunities now, but you won't have them forever.

Get off your butt to do the things you've always promised yourself; and do whatever it takes to get your adrenaline racing and put the twinkle back in your eye. Pledge to let go of any or all situations that are compromising your flirt-appeal. Make that well-overdue career change, living adjustment or just get rid of that awful friend, and lose that haunted, stooped over look, the one that translates to a "Kick Me" sign stuck to your back! Embrace your party-pants plan, celebrate your single life – learn to spin a hula-hoop for god's sake. And take Andy Warhol's advice to "make your own luck."

Whatever you do – don't waste time sitting around waiting for Boy Wonder to waltz up! He'll only appear when you're keeping yourself flirty, quirky and perky. Truly it's Sod's Law.


*"I was never the skinniest, the prettiest or the smartest,*

*but I tried the hardest."*

- Helen Gurley Brown, founder American *Cosmopolitan*

## *Step 3*
## *7-Day-Fill-Out-and-Keep-Flirt-Plan*

*Day 1.* Sort out your life: Organise! Clear! Declutter!

*Day 2.* The makings of Action Diva.

*Day 3.* Getting in touch with your Inner Kid.

*Day 4.* Unleashing your Dare-Devil Diva.

*Day 5.* From Workaholic to Weekend Warrior.

*Day 6.* Adventure Diva.

*Day 7.* Travel Diva.

# DAY 1
## OCD: ORGANISE! CLEAR! DECLUTTER!

First things first. It's time to get your life sorted out, so let's start with the basics. Ensure your living space is clean, organised and ready for action. You know what they say, a clean living space equals a clean mind, so let's make a plan to get yours in order. Create a quiet, calm place from which you can plot, plan and scheme your way to *Sex And The City* divadom. *Ladies prepare your station!*

Don't get put off by thinking you will lose a weekend of your life doing this, or any party time at all, because you won't. Just put aside an hour a day for a week or two and attack one section at a time, it's more manageable and less frustrating. Take advantage of those days when you're just not in the mood to face the world – stay in and sort out the cupboards instead. It may not seem very Flirt Diva-ish at the time, but you'll be loving the results as you zoom zoom from room to room, especially when you get to treat yourself with shiny, new things to decorate all that extra space you've created.

### First stop, the boudoir:

It goes without saying your boudoir should be sparkling, shiny and all sexed up – ready for any impromptu adventures! So the first task is a good tidy and clean out – don't yawn this is important! Especially when you see the calming effects of a quick declutter, and more if you're inspired to create your own Flirt-Shui Love Corner. Interested? OK, here's what the experts recommend. Firstly they say it should be positioned on the far right hand side as you walk into your room.

117

*Here's what you'll need.*

1. A brightly coloured back-lit wall
2. An image of your favourite decorative image
3. Fresh flowers to energise your sleeping space
4. Your favourite mementos
5. Scented candles

Now illuminate your decorative image, light the scented candles and dedicate a shrine to your newly developing confidence; it could be a photo-album, scrap-book, or a hat-box collection of your best ever memories in the form of mementos, awards, favourite poems, letters, affirmations – anything and everything that acts as a reminder of the person you love being and reflects your place as the Queen of Fabulousness! Look at it last thing each night before going to sleep and repeat your *Vamp Mantra. I am Action Diva!*

Next, move along to the wardrobe. If it's been in play-it-safe-mode for far too long, and badly in need of transformation, do it now. Prune it back, tidy it up and revamp it, ready for action. Host "Swap Evenings" where you crack open a couple of bottles of wine and exchange your unwanted clothes. Out with the old and in with the new.

Now look at all your bits and bobs, do they need sorting? If so, start with your accessories, there's nothing worse than faffing around looking for your favourite earrings and silver winkle-pickers when you're running late! Have everything ready to go, go, go at a moment's notice. The point is there will be no more lame excuses for not going out, because, "I couldn't find anything to wear!"

Rejuvenate the bathroom; re-organise your toiletries and make-up bag so that any old stale products are refreshed and replenished. Putting rotting make-up on your face is like rubbing dirt into it. It's not good.

Everything should be tidied up, acting as an incentive to get glammed up at a moment's notice, on any given night. And when you're ready, get out there for a big night and go mad. Even better, invite somebody back to yours. Mr Bloody Marvellous won't know what hit him.

Finally, get stuck into all your admin. Yes I know it's boring, but it's impossible to focus on yourself when you've got an anxiety disorder about, well, everything! So hop to it. Don't take it on all in one go, tackle it one thing at a time over the course of a week, or a month, to get the bulk of it done. Write a list and lock it down. Make those medical appointments, do the banking, the ironing, the filing. Confront that pile of bills and ring your mum damn you! Attack the stuff that's weighing you down rather than letting it suck up any more negative energy. Only then will you start feeling the full effects of Flirt Divadom. And then sit back and let the party to begin.

# DAY 2

## THE MAKING OF AN ACTION DIVA

So now that you've got the humdrum stuff out of the way, it's time to plan the fun bits. This is where you get a taste to do the things that float your boat, whether it's glam, glitz or grungy good times.

If you live in a big city, there's a world of drama and imagination outside the mainstream just waiting to be unearthed – if you're prepared to look for it that is. Avoid "Club Wotever" with its self-conscious scene; hanging around places like that won't do you any favours. Pick somewhere fabulous instead – not somewhere all fake and posy, but somewhere where *you can be fabulous*. There are so many themed bars and clubs about, it's easy to find one that brings out the best in you. Walk into the club and own it. Being cool is old hat. Having fun is the new black. Even cooler than thou Kate Moss dresses up for '80s nights at various clubs around London and dances around looking like a twat. Good god!

Think big. Think party with the Glitterati. Prepare for a fashion upgrade to show off at some fancy schmancy ball with corsets and diamonds. Watch everyone bounce, spin, twirl and delight in the art of the flirt. Jump aboard the pop express and glitter ball through the disco infected world of fun. Get your hands dirty, decadent, and lustful. The point is, have a change of scene. Anything, so long as it's different!

Think of your big night out with humour. Use comic fantasy if it helps, or be even more daring and create an alter ego. Imagine you're starring as the hot babe superhero. An exotic beauty, or Madame Lash gearing up for a pash. Do something, do anything, but for-the-love-of-god, don't sit at home moping. This is your research. Say yes to every invitation, initiate your own events, get out there and watch, learn, observe!

Make a habit of treating yourself. Learn to live with happiness and gluttony. Become a gourmet guru or an armchair foodie and go to Gastronomic Trivia nights. Get all dressed up and book yourself in for a swanky dinner with champagne and desert somewhere fab. Or nail the art of making something you will be really proud of, whether that's a seafood bouillabaisse, sushi, Swedish meatballs or just a curry in a hurry. Swill wine in the name of being a connoisseur. You're probably already a barstool junkie, so why not go the whole hog and actually sign up for bar-school? Do a class in mixology and create your own signature cocktail – added bonus this *will* make you popular with the blokes!

> *Golden Rule: It's all about having the time of your life, not meeting the love of your life! Stop operating out of emergency mode and take the time to prepare!*

## DAY 3
## GET IN TOUCH WITH YOUR INNER KID

As Einstein said, "Imagination is more important than knowledge". So tap into your inner juvenile-delinquent to get your adrenalin pumping. Gear up your Flirt Squad and list the things you loved doing as kids, then organise a day spent doing it. And don't try to be cool. The point is to be as goofy as you can!

So do anything – play hide 'n' seek, hopscotch or have a treasure hunt. Whirl through an energetic session of rollerblading, ice skating or table tennis. Spend an afternoon body surfing, horse-riding or go-kart riding. Play board games, twister or hopscotch. Take off for a weekend of camping; hiking or a caravan trip. Prepare an afternoon picnic or a fishing trip or host an Alice in Wonderland style garden tea party. Just do something, anything kiddy-ish and fun.

# DAY 4

## UNLEASH YOUR DARE DEVIL DIVA

The simple act of learning something new has the power to give you mystery, depth and intrigue. You'll be the one who gets out there and actually does it, while everyone else just sits around talking about it.

This is the time to think about your hidden talent. It's no good having talent if you don't know what to do with it! Stretch your imagination. Create something artistic that's truly and originally yours. Make your own T-shirt slogan, jewellery, accessories, anything cool and crafty. Play poker and learn the art of how to read people. Throw a hula-hoop party and grow delicious edible things in your garden.

**Some ideas to get you started:**

1.  Replace watching reruns of *X-Factor* with:

    *Brazilian dance or Viennese Waltz lessons*

2.  Replace hanging out with the same friends every Friday and Saturday night with:

    *Joining a new group and networking your head off*

3.  Replace watching trash TV with:

    *Trying your hand at still life drawing as a student or as a model.*

4.  Replace buying gifts and getting ripped off with:

    *Making them with your own fair hands*

**Now use your imagination to come up with 3 hobbies you'd like to try:**

    1.

    2.

    3.


**Fancy some paranormal fun with good old fashioned gobbledygook?**
Find out what your future holds with a reading in: Numerology, tarot, psychic, tea leaves, palm or face reading.


## Dare Devil Diva

They say that fear is the very thing that rocks us to the core and makes us value life. I'm not saying you have to become a Jujitsu enthusiast or a professional gladiator, but having a personality transplant does require a lot of *doing* on your part. Take the plunge and book in for that something you've always wanted to do but never had the nerve. Did you see that episode of *Sex And The City* where Carrie takes trapeze lessons? That's what I'm talking about! Start off with baby steps to find your own personal adrenalin thrill. As well as having the time of your life, you'll turn yourself into the energizer bunny. Your audience will lap up your stories and be inspired by the fact that you're up for surfing, sushi, salsa, scuba diving, or anything stimulating starting with an 's'!

**Think you can handle the rough and tumble of any of the following?**

 Bungee jumping

 Go-carting

 Juggling

 Riding a chopper bike

 Signing up for stunt school

 Sword fighting

**What are 3 things you've *always* wanted to do?**

 1.

 2.

 3.

**Get a culture injection:**

Get your head around some new and interesting stuff. Visit an art gallery, museum or an exhibition. See as many different shows as you can! Check out your local theatres or town hall for concerts and performances. Visit a sex museum for saucy topics to throw out there and shake up an otherwise staid conversation. Anything as long as it's different to what you normally do!

## *DAY 5*

## *FROM WORKAHOLIC TO WEEKEND WARRIOR*

Ah the meaning of work. Like all addictions, work has its price. Have a good honest look at the job, or career you're in, and ask yourself if it's really and truly right for you. It's heartbreaking how long we can spend in soul destroying jobs – and hey, I should know! If disillusionment or frustration in your job, or your career has taken its toll, it's time to do something about it.

**Set yourself a 90 day career-plan:**
If you're planning a career change anytime soon and fancy yourself queen of Success and Money – or the S & M Queen – a 90-day plan will give you plenty of time to whack your CV into shape, get yourself registered at various recruitment agencies and see what's out there in job land. If you really want to be smart though, use your spare time to invest in a mini-course and develop another skill-set. That way you'll never be caught short and you'll always have a contingency plan. This is from someone who changed paths mid-career because – life's too short.

*"Nothing is permanent and things either go up or they go down. It's your luck to be given the ball, and you'd better keep it bouncing."*
- Joan Rivers

## DAY 6

## ADVENTURE DIVA

Go wild in the jungle! Or the zoo will do if there's no jungle handy. Better still, a forest or the National Park. It doesn't really matter where you go, so long as you're out amongst nature and enjoying a different scene. Become a self-appointed ambassador for your cause and do your bit to save an endangered species – tigers, gorillas – donkeys!

### Get some air in you hair

- Get out in the country air and do your best Annie Oakley sharpshooter impersonation.

- Muck in with a weekend campathon.

- Book in for beachside boot-camp.

- Adopt an orang-utan or a panda, a labra doodle – any animal at all.

- Grow "love herbs" like basil or sage, rosemary or thyme.

- Hit the slopes (real or fake) for some skiing.

- Get your skates on!

- Go fishing

**Or, just indulge in your guilty pleasures. What's your Top 3?**

1................................................................................

2................................................................................

3................................................................................

## DAY 7
## *TRAVEL DIVA*

If you've always wanted to travel abroad, or just get away for a mini-break, but found that you keep putting it on the back-burner, now is the time to start planning. You won't be single for ever, so lock down the fantasy stuff to do now!

Thanks to the internet bringing the world closer together, it's easy to be a globetrotter and organise to meet online friends anywhere abroad. So why not do it? Travelling alone doesn't have to be lonely; there are loads of well thought out opportunities available for singles, and provided you follow safety precautions, it can be the adventure of a lifetime.

Imagine how fab it would be to go somewhere exotic and cavort with the colourful locals at the drop of a hat? Even better if you get around to learning the lingo, familiarising yourself with the local cuisine, or picking up some useful info about the local culture before you go. Beg, borrow or steal a video camera and make your debut feature travel documentary. Use it as another opportunity to give your chat skills a work out. Foreigners are no different to locals, they love talking about themselves too. Ask just one question, about their lives, their country and in most places, you will slot in like you belong.

So, lovely lady, what are you waiting for? Book that trip and hop on that plane, train or automobile. Of course there is always a very good chance that you may luck out with a sizzling holiday romance, perhaps with someone whose first language is not English, ooh la la! All well and good – except – it pays to keep in mind that there are different rules about flirting everywhere in the world. You will encounter specific local customs that you will need to pay attention to. Especially since flirting rituals change dramatically from country to country.

### Reality check – this ain't no fairytale

Courtship patterns within the Western world are all fairly interchangeable, but that's not the case everywhere. Rather frighteningly, flirting has actually been banned in some Asian countries and offenders, both local and international, have been known to be jailed for inappropriate behaviour! So please remember that anti-flirting laws are alive and well in various parts of the world. And yes it does seem odd since most Westernized countries are flocking to flirting like ducks to water, but each to their own. Ultimately it is our responsibility to be respectful of local customs and abide by the rules – or face the consequences.

So in the event that you do find yourself having a raunchy old time when you visit a new country, you might want to familiarise yourself with their customs before you go, so you don't cause any offence or court any unnecessary controversy, or in the worst case scenario, go to jail!

### Number One Flirting Abroad Tip:

*#1 Rule: When in Dubai do not have sex on the beach.*
*#2 Rule: Do not attempt to flirt with the local officials.*
Remember the British couple arrested for doing more than frolicking on the beach in Dubai? Don't be coming unstuck like that!

*"I was born and bred to be a great flirt. I'm Southern – it's in my blood. We don't take it too seriously down South – it's a form of social relating that has nothing to do with sex. Which can make it dangerous when you travel."*
- Cybil Shepherd, U.S. actress

### *Flirt Review: Finding your Signature Flirt Profile*

Now that you've unleashed your Action Diva and seen how your quality of life can benefit dramatically from an energy overhaul, you're in the perfect position to draw up a social timetable which will thrust you into frenzied new flirt-zones.

So, under the heading Step 3, list any creative ideas you have for exciting new ways you can keep on jazzing up your life. This is fantasy fulfilment stuff, so write it all down. Describe your dream life and the adventures you would have. The thrills and spills you would love to come your way? How will you bring the wow-factor into your life and how will you keep it? Don't hold back; let your imagination run wild.

Finally write a few words about what you can do, in both the short and long term, to sustain this dynamic new lifestyle and keep it fizzing.

# Congratulations you've completed your Step 3 missions!

## Step 3 Learning Outcomes

### *Key points*

> ➤ Do whatever it takes to get that adrenalin going.
>
> ➤ Be comfortable in your own skin.
>
> ➤ Create and design your own T-shirt slogan for life.
>
> ➤ Work your charm from the minute you leave the house.

### *Checklist*

- ✓ Curiosity
- ✓ Lust for Life
- ✓ Passion

*Vamp Mantra: Lights, Camera, Action!*

Finally ALWAYS follow the 3 Golden rules of flirt divadom:

1. *Leave the House!*
2. *Leave the House!*
3. *Leave the House!*

# Step 4. Glamarazzi: How to glam up like a Flirt Diva

*Week 4*

This week's focus is all about the physical you: Your body image and how you feel about it. Here's where you'll start to think about exiting new ways to overhaul your entire image, and gain more confidence about the way you look and feel. It's all about feeling and looking fresher when you step out as we crack out the Glam It Up Seven-day makeover plan and activate your Get-Out-Of-Couch-Potato-Land card.

**Key phrase:** *Personal image*

**Challenge**: *To make daily improvements*

**Goal**: *Be prepared for any occasion*

**Result:** *Feeling hot, hot, hot!*

### *Chapter 6. From Blah to Bombshell*

As we strut and sashay our way through this section, we'll study the looks and shapes of some of our most photographed icons, and consider ways to adapt the bits that suit you. I'll be campaigning against beauty trends and cheering you on to get your own personal diva fever going on. It's fine to be inspired, just so long as we don't become slaves to the trends, or big copy-cats who lack spirit or originality

So it's time to peek into the looking glass to see how your sense of style and body image fits into all this. Because if looks or beauty issues are cramping your style, you need to do something about it pronto. That means getting your head out of the Hall of Lame and into the Hall of Fame.

Whatever your size or shape, it just takes a little know-how to turn drizzle to sizzle; stressed to best dressed; homely to honey-pie. Take what's there and enhance it. Make the most of your gorgeous figure and individual style. You may not be getting whisked off for drinks at Bungalow 8 tonight but that doesn't mean you can't make a big Flirt Diva splash at your local!

The only way to go from frazzled to dazzled is to start with a complete glam over and honey, you're going to get the works! Keep reading for the complete low-down on all things glam and body passion – unless you're in the point one-percent of the population who is perfect already? If so you can skip the rest of this chapter but, if you're like the rest of us, plagued with doubt and confusion about the baffling mysteries of modern beauty – keep reading!

We all know it can it can be easy to forget about the trivial stuff, like you know, looking hot. Especially at the end of the long, exhausting day when there are so many other things to get stressed about. But there's no excuse for us Flirt Divas not to look our best. And why shouldn't we? Yes, we get that being a babe magnet is not about having perfect bone structure, but it is about making an effort. We can't all be natural beauties but we can make the most of our hair, skin and clothes.

Plan your preparation with meticulous attention and the rest will follow. That means making the most of what you've got. Be the poster-girl for Real Beauty versus the Airbrushed bollocks. Raise the bar. Channel your inner goddess. Dedicate yourself to grooming, hygiene, minty breath and feeling comfortable in your own skin. Develop your signature look and stick with it. We're not talking military operation, just organised calm instead of outright chaos.

This Flirt Diva remembers taking one of those hideous 6.00am Easyjet flights not so long ago, you know the ones, where your alarm is set for stupid o'clock, and you fall out of bed at 3.30am. You make your way groggily to the bathroom, wishing you hadn't sloshed over to the bar and bought that third bottle of Rosé at "final drinks" last night! You look in the mirror, nearly gagging at the vision that looks back at you, but eventually stumble out the door with horrendous hair and blotchy bare faced chic – except there's nothing chic about it! You scramble into the fluorescent clinical madness that is the airport and that's when you see her – that impeccable couture princess. Teetering along in kitten heels, snug jeans and cashmere sweater, perfect hair framing her impeccably made-up face, all set off by her Gucci bags and Louis Vuitton luggage. You just gawp at her, and sink a little lower in your despair as you try to hitch last season's low-slung jeans over your builders' bum crack, thinking, "Why dear lord, can't that be me?" But it can!


***Babes, bombshells and bimbos***

And let's face it ladies, in the absence of a man, personal maintenance can become somewhat relaxed. Who hasn't gone out on the town with fat sucking undies and an exploding mine of shame lurking under their Topshop frock – hmmmm? But thanks to the Flirt Diva revolution – that won't be happening any more!

The aspiring Flirt Diva must be prepared for *anything* – that's the point. And today more than ever, we really need to step things up a notch. Especially with the intriguing newsflash that today's modern male is more vain than ever. *According to a British Poll, men are spending up to 28 minutes on grooming – which is up by 30% in five years.* ♥ Watch out girls! And while we might appreciate a man who makes a little effort, we don't really want to be stuck with a buffoon who spends his whole day preening, posing and peacocking!

Certainly the metrosexualisation of men has ensured they either use, or are at the very least, *aware* of, moisturizers, body deodorants, hair grooming products and even make-up for men. "Oi, care for some guyliner or manscara?" Why should Russell Brand be the only one who gets to wear it? There's also a rumour that men have taken to wearing `mirdles' (man girdles), `mantypose' (you guessed it, pantyhose for men) and `mankinis' (take a bow Borat). Recently P. Diddy took it upon himself to tell us: "Men owe it to women to ensure they're well groomed. I wax my privates. " ♥♥ Too much information thanks!

The world of glamour and beauty is addictive, compelling, maddening and expensive. The marketing gurus behind the make-up, hair and perfume brands are conspiring to make celebrities the richest women on the planet by selling a slice of their sex appeal. That's why we're studying them with a voracious appetite. We want to see the dividends for looking so damn sexy. We may not always approve of their romantic lives, but by god,

---

♥ Revealed in a poll by grooming brand *Bulldog*
♥♥ London Paper, June 16, 2008

we're watching! And whether we realise it or not, we're picking up the tips and tricks along the way. Step 4 all about using that influence in a positive and healthy way.

The message is – keep up! I'll be the first to 'fess up. I've spent too many long days and nights tap, tap, tapping away at my computer on some never ending deadline, clad in jeans and an old t-shirt, feeling like the most pathetically groomed woman on the planet. It's those days where the simple task of arranging myself for a big night out, or, gasp, A Date, has seemed as daunting a mission as any. The old one-step-forward-two-steps-back rhythm of the wax/exfoliate/ moisturize/mani/pedi/ blow-dry boogie can seemingly take over your life! *If* you're not keeping up with regular maintenance.

There is an art to keeping up with the frenzied cycle of body grooming in diva-sized bits, and there are two ways to approach it. You can either squeeze it into your life begrudgingly, or you can embrace it! Keep in mind that being at one with your body instinctively puts you in touch with your self-esteem. Making a go of putting on a special outfit, or experimenting with some fun new make-up is like honouring an inner dignity that we have within ourselves, it makes us look better, but just as importantly, it makes us *feel* better!

But that doesn't stop us from wanting to wake up beautiful! Who hasn't had that fantasy? And it's harmless enough, but we do have to get over the idea that beauty or physical perfection can make us happy, it's just not true! As for those airbrushed images of perfection staring out at us from the pages of magazines, they're not real – they're just pretend.

Who in Hollywood A-list circles hasn't enhanced, tweaked, whitened, brightened or Botox-ed something? It might make them look better, but as we've discovered, Having More Beauty doesn't strengthen *anyone's* chances of living the Happy Ever After.

## *Chapter 7. From lipstick to lingerie*

It's useful to be realistic about the cards you were dealt in terms of your physical appearance – just be honest about it. You have your list of "best qualities" from Step 1 to go back and refer to, so now that you've identified your best assets, it's time to accentuate them. You've also got your Flirt Squad around to remind you of your best qualities, so really you should start to see new lashings of confidence sprouting up very soon!

You might be surprised at how a bit of effort can make up for what you lack in the classic beauty stakes. And frankly, unless you're a supermodel, the only way to look continuously gorgeous is to put in the effort. The trick is to say goodbye to *too* many late nights and Really Bad Habits. From there you can sass, rattle and shimmy your style into the super Flirt Diva stratosphere. You might not have Naomi Campbell's insolent bum, or Cameron Diaz-tastic thighs, but that doesn't mean you can't focus on your best assets and `work it!' Start now. Defog the mirror and study the characteristics that make you the unique and exceptional, individual that you are. *Viva la diva!*

And yes, a lot of the results are somewhat in the mind – you already *know* you're going to look and feel better when you wake up after a good night's sleep. It's the sense of relief you get when your well-rested, well-moisturised image smiles back at you in the mirror. That's the reward and it starts the day with a buzz. It's the same with diet, somehow, miraculously, if you lay off the junk food and the booze for a while, the improvement can be incredible.

For the moment, the secret weapons are those things that are attainable. Sparkly eyes, soft, dewy skin, shiny hair and silky lingerie, a cool, fizzy tonic for the ego. Pretty things that give you the secret knowledge you're ready for anything – should the flirt-ortunity present itself.

You could argue that there is more to life than the adroit application of fire-engine red lipstick and good hair days, but we all know it's not true! It is important to have our trusted beauty tools at our fingertips and polish up a trademark look that's easily applied, anytime and anywhere. It's just a shame it doesn't always work in practise. We've all been guilty of turning up somewhere unprepared, looking our most crap and Sod's Law – bumping into that someone special.

Let me be clear though, the society of Flirt Divas are not demanding that you step out of the door with a full face of war paint. But we are talking about religiously adhering to the Bad-Gal-Lashes-and-Shiny-Lips-Brigade – no handbag should ever be without mascara and lip-gloss. Make no mistake these are the most vital tools of the trade, and I'm sorry but unless you're Angelina Jolie – they're important. They form the basis of our daily uniform and steel us for the experience of stepping out with enough cockiness to face the battle. Whether you're a student, or a hot-shot executive, the simple art of looking fresh and alert will help renew your confidence and put you ahead of the competition. So long as you're not obsessive about it of course.

And it really is the simple things. Mascara makes sleepy eyes sparkle, beady eyes big and puffy eyes pristine. It cures depression, fuels love rivals – and ends wars. It's magic stuff. It costs nothing to have the best lashes in town. The best mascara is also the cheapest, Maybelline, as used by all the supermodels. Apply it with tender loving care. Twenty five lashes for each eye. Not a stroke less! Let it smudge, swoop, smudge and swoosh. Let it frame and fan your eyes. Let it snort in the face of bare faced chic and shout out Fun! Mischief! Minx! Use your lashes to have another drink and go and chat with that chappy. Go on!

139

Even the most superb bone structure can be let down by a "tired" look when there's no emphasis or colour to highlight the bone definitions, eyes or lips. For this Flirt Diva, it's a professional choice over and above anything. Just think in terms of really basic flirting – how are you supposed to indulge if you can't perform lash-aerobics?

While you're on your way to getting gorgeous, remember, the most striking girls are not necessarily the prettiest – but the most interesting. I'm thinking of the Professional Cool Girls, like Chloe Sevigny, Sarah Jessica Parker, Lily Allen, America Ferrera and Kelly Osborne amongst others. The common link here is their quirky sense of style, not their conventional looks. Anyone who invests a chunk of serious time and commitment can get themselves a slice of that. Victoria Beckham has been brave enough (or honest enough) to acknowledge she owes more to meticulous grooming than genetics for her look (love it or loathe it). Despite the trophy husband and her ability to be perennial paparazzi favourite – the former Spice Girl insists she doesn't consider herself exceptionally attractive. She told *Allure* magazine: "I'm a normal-looking girl, and I just make the best of what I have. I'm incredibly ordinary."

### Shimmy your style into the super diva stratosphere

Indeed some of the most divatastic celebrities on the planet are big enough to admit that they're not the prettiest, but they've got the moves, the style, the signature red-hot lips and the attitude. As we've already established, these girls do have A-grade access to world class advice on everything from image and diet to voice training and rigorous personal coaching – this is what makes them the masters – which is why it makes sense to be led by their style and approach. They are the absolute experts when it comes to putting it altogether – along with an army of stylists, beauticians, therapists and various other magic types or course!

So why not take some lessons? See what it feels like to be impeccably turned out like Dita, Christina or Gwen; or to have Madonna's yogified body, J Lo's booty or Beyoncé's bling. So what if it's unlikely that we'll ever have the jet-setting lives, eye popping wardrobes, personal stylists, live-in hairdressers, or bulging beauty budgets. There's no harm in sprinkling a little stardust into our lives to improve our chances of going to the ball is there?

We know that conventional good looks aren't everything – but you might be surprised by what you can achieve with an overhaul. And look on the bright side, nobody appreciates a beautiful face if its only expression is a sour one that looks like it's just been bitch slapped. Bottom line: you don't have to be a whippet thin model, or a classic beauty, so long as your appearance is happening enough to reveal a clean, shiny-haired, fully functioning human being.

Going overboard can be just as bad. Girls that look insanely sickeningly good don't look that way by accident. They're obsessed with it, sad little narcissists that they are! Inspecting themselves furiously in the magnifying glasses, double and triple checking their image; taking Polaroids before they step out for god's sake! Never believing that the mirror tells the whole truth and only photo evidence will do! There's a price to pay for this level of vanity which eats up hours and hours of getting ready time – playtime is over before you even get to the ball.

### Babe Magnify yourself (and celebrate your natural beauty)

You see this Flirt Diva wasn't always so fabulous. Moving to London in 2005 meant starting all over again and doing the grind, in a day job that nearly destroyed my happiness and most certainly my mind.

After slumming it for way too long, it was high time to get my old self back. I decided to take matters into my own hands. It was time for a change. In New York the presidential candidates were slogging it out; in Paris the riots were breaking out, but I had more pressing matters to attend to – ladies, the transformation from gargoyle to glamazon had begun.

As I redecorated my bedroom and refurbished my dreams, I looked to sex bombs like the immaculate Dita Von Teese for inspiration. I wanted to kick-start my va va voom process and feel like a woman again. Looks weren't the most important thing by a long shot, but I still knew what I knew. It was time to bring out the big guns. It was time to work it! There was one mother of a life change coming my way and I wanted to be the best I could.

*"Office worker sheds dowdy day job to star as burlesque bombshell".*

And why shouldn't I treat myself? I have the same interests as you – I want my skin to glow, my health to show and my thighs not to wobble. I want the *Sex and the City* factor. I want to flounce over to the mirror for reassurance and know that I'm doing OK: "Mirror Mirror on the wall, am I even, like, moderately attractive?" 'Yes!' it would holler. "Well thank heavens for that!" I would sigh and laugh, breathing out *without* popping my trouser buttons. And I would relax, refusing to let my fat, fugly days interfere with my ability to face the world.

And for the most part, I am prepared to work at it. I think a lot about body issues – it's hard not to when ravishing, ravenous superstars are shoved down your throat 24/7 isn't it? Do I think I'll ever live up that image? No! Do I want to? Hell no! We already know that airbrushing is de rigour and the images we see in magazines are bollocks. It's a ploy designed to make us feel inadequate, but I'm OK. I've got my own style going on thanks.

Or do I?

I decided that in the name of the research and in the best interests of Flirt Divadom, I needed to lift my game a notch and practice what I preach. Yeah baby. I would get out there and sample every affordable beauty queen dream – you can call it a perk of the job, I call it survival.

Indulge me in this fantasy if you will. I would electrify my bleak, black wardrobe, stake out chichi boutiques, made- to-measure Louboutin heels and flowing, Swarovski beaded emerald frocks, just like the one Kate Moss wore to the *Fashion Rocks* gala. I would visit my favourite clothing store and get my own *Glam Squad*. I would snaffle up this season's must have cropped leather jacket, fabulous vintage Jacqui O sunglasses, and step out in fashion-forward spiky stiletto shoe boots with my Balenciaga-inspired pooch purse.

I would experiment with clip-in Pammy Anderson style hair extensions, spray tans, eyelash perms and blushes with names like *Orgasm*. I would take to wearing an undersized Chloe bag and carrying a Paris Hilton style Chihuahua named Foo-Foo. Oh to be so gloriously shallow.

The only problem is, ahem, I'm not really that sort of girly girl. And I certainly don't have the blow-out budget – so, back to reality. I would kick-start my reinvention with the very basics that nature provided: a sensible diet, rigorous cleanse, tone and moisturiser routine, a healthy life-style and boot camp fitness regime. With my hourglass credentials intact (always nicer than thinking of oneself as a sugar-plump fairy), I would enter into the, "Unleash my Warrior Diva" zone.

After exploring my options – I could skate, swim or shimmy – Shakira style – to fitness. Or, I could strip as it turned out, with Carmen Electra's *Stripper-robics*, the benefit being that I could practice at home. And sure I might look like a total twat, but you must admit, exercise soaked in genuine Hollywood sex-appeal does make it more exotic!

I would vow to get up one hour earlier every morning to redistribute the newly formed love handles that had taken up residence on my being over Christmas, and work on my body language and posture while analysing every aspect of my physical behaviour. Could I walk elegantly in heels? Did I move with confidence? Was I slouching? Could I improve my posture? Or rid myself of `computer slump'?

I would keep my chin raised slightly for a crisp, clean profile and study the science of curve-ology in relation to my height, mindset and body weight. Whilst I had long ago accepted that being size 12 was hoochy cool, I knew it wouldn't hurt to tone up a tad. I could feel my booty billowing out behind me so I looked to the fashionistas for advice: *"You can look at your big arse two ways"* they declared. *"Either hide it, or celebrate it."* I decided to celebrate it by opening two bottles of bubbly – one for each cheek.

Failing that I would bring in the plastic surgeons – I'm kidding! It's got zero to do with plastic fantastic looks. Well unless your name is Katie Price who shakes her St. Tropez-ed ass and says: "I would rather have a designer body than a designer outfit. Luckily, I can afford both."
*Boob Flash to Jordan: Beauty is confidence. Not a bum lift*

Bottom line if you're an aspiring Flirt Diva, it's part of the gig to look your best. The good news is you don't have to spend a fortune or dedicate hours of your life to the pursuit of beauty – but you do need a routine. You also have to believe that whatever time and effort you put in will be rewarded with amazing results.

These are the foundations when it comes to schmoozing and cruising and making the best impressions. It's all important stuff, especially since we know only too well that our body issues can and often do, screw up the way we see ourselves and present ourselves. The way you look is a barometer of your inner self – remember that. And when you stride onto the field and honey, you will be on fire! But not before you've glammed up and pranced in front of the mirror and whooped, "Whoa. I look hot!" So throw those shoulders back, walk that diva walk, talk the diva talk and strap yourself into your Flirt Divamobiles, and hang on for the ride.

## *Step 4*

## *7-Day-Fill-Out-and-Keep-Flirt-Plan*

*Day 1.* List your Beauty and Style Heroes

*Day 2*. Have a Pamper Day

*Day 3.* Do something Naughty but Nice

*Day 4.* Glow with Good Health

*Day 5.* Get the Dita Von Teese Look-at-Me posture

*Day 6.* Book a Makeover Session

*Day 7.* Complete the Glam Quiz

# DAY 1
## LIST YOUR BEAUTY AND STYLE HEROES

You already know the women that inspire you in the general sense, now it's time to identify those whose beauty style appeals and narrow it down. Who are your style icons? What is their look? How can you get it?

Refer back to the glossies for inspiration. Spend time at the library and flick through beautifully illustrated fashion books. Describe the look of the women you admire in as much detail as you can. Get right down to the nitty gritty. You can have as many different influences as you like. I have mascara influences which of course I will bore you with. Audrey Hepburn – all time queen of the lashes. Winona Ryder, Penelope Cruz. Keira Knightley. Natalie Imbruglia. Cheryl Cole – I don't see why they should be superior to me in their application of bad gal lashes!

Think about the changes you need to make to revamp your style. Consider the ways that you can change, improve or tweak *your* overall look. Once you've done that, work on focusing it down to a style that you can call your very own.

Taking inspiration from your beauty heroes and adapting it to your own look, personality and style is a great starting point. *Provided you don't take it too seriously and end up going under the scalpel's knife to get a "celebrity look!" Sadly some women are going that far to imitate the look of their fave idols, desperate to "be them". And the scary thing is, they can, provided they've got the cash, the desire and the stomach for it!*

Your style idols don't have to be high profile either. I'll never forget one of mine. She was a real life Business Barbie, working for my parent's as their office manager when I was a teen. She was as slim as a whippet,

147

effortlessly sleek and always the style icon, never kitted out in anything less than the most chic designer garb. She strode around in great trench coats with bold, patent heels and charcoal grey pencil skirts. She had the most glistening blue-black bob and porcelain complexion and her lashes were like nothing I'd ever seen before, long, luxurious – just spellbinding. She taught me the importance of image, presentation and dressing for success, and made me appreciate how it could make you look like a goddamn celebrity. Perhaps not surprisingly she went on to become the uber stylish wife of a big name media personality. It's true what they say – dress for success, and you will attract it.

*Flirt Alert*: Don't emulate the style of a celebrity whose body shape you simply don't have!

*"I make a point to never, ever point out my physical flaws ... this is advice I give to women as often as I can. People don't notice the things we see in ourselves that we hate, so why direct them to it? Living with your flaws doesn't mean you should tell people about them."*

- Dita Von Teese

# DAY 2
## HAVE A PAMPER DAY

It's completely personal how you approach the whole beauty extravaganza. You can either go all out and spend the day getting pampered at a day-spa or an exotic bathhouse – nothing will make you feel more rejuvenated than lounging around for a few hours before going home to lie back in your little flirt-pod!  Alternatively you can forget about spending all your hard earned pennies at the salon and try your hand at DIY style beauty. Give yourself an overhaul with the works; include your own "spa therapy" complete with a deluxe exfoliation and full body wrap. Whichever way you do it, if you commit to at least one feel good/look good treat every week you will get amazing results. The motivation need simply be to hatch a plan which will have you looking and feeling like the Queen of Sheba every time you leave the house.

***Tips for keeping up the frenzied cycle of body grooming and maintenance***
Key rules: smile, glide and keep your cool.

- Make advance beauty arrangements so you're never caught unawares or unprepared!
- Aim for Real Beauty Vs the airbrushed look.
- Change your perfume regularly.
- Have at least one day a month of top-to-toe primping, preening and pampering.
- Get a massage – revel in that touchy-feely-feel-good therapy.
- Tanorexia – don't ever wear the damaging effects of the sun's rays when you can fake it.

- Let your hair luxuriate with a deep conditioning treatment and colour (and keep up the good work with your own at-home conditioning treatments in-between appointments.)
- Book a DIY styling session – where the stylist actually teaches you how to maintain the look at home in-between salon visits.
- Treat yourself to a "do" for a big event. Go for an upsweep, a dramatic new look, a totally wild new hair colour or some good old fashioned curl power!

Star Hollywood reporter Perez Hilton insists that: *"Women want to see other women looking not so great. A shot of someone's armpit hair or cellulite sells more than a lovely, set-up, airbrushed pic"*.

Ha-ha-ha! We gleefully squeal.

"So you're not so perfect after all, 'ey bitch!"

*"I'm on the `I'm going to drink loads of wine and eat what I like diet. My body is my body, I'm perfectly happy with it and if everyone else isn't, that's there problem. Check out my arms, they wobble.'"*
- Lily Allen: *Grazia Magazine*

# DAY 3
## DO SOMETHING NAUGHTY BUT NICE

Transform yourself with a look that you've always aspired to, but never been brave enough to try. Do something radical and exotic – whether that's a piercing, tattoo or a designer bikini wax – there are a mind-boggling amount of shapes and colours to choose from! Go incognito for a day with a wash-out crazy hair colour or a clip on waist-length hairpiece. Have some fun with a temporary tattoo; coloured eye-contacts; eyelash extensions or a false beauty spot a la Cindy Crawford.

Become a hardcore hedonist dress-up queen, unleash your goddess of seduction and channel your inner burlesque belle. Bathe yourself in milk and honey and clad yourself in something slinky; channel the glamour puss that is Dita Von Teese. And listen to her when she says: *"wearing stockings every day will change your life"*. Invest in a blood red lipstick, corset, suspenders, garter belt and 5 inch heels. Miaow!

Doing something racy and a little risqué could lead you to all sorts of adventures, but you'll never know unless you try.

*"I don't wake up like Cindy Crawford I morph into her."*
– Supermodel Cindy Crawford at the top of her supermodel fame.

# DAY 4
## ADDRESS YOUR BODY ISSUES

It's time to find new ways to get fit and fight flab. This is where you get together with your Flirt-Squad for some serious physical exertion and work it – instead of sitting in the pub downing a week's worth of calorific cocktails!

Make this your time to strive for a healthier diet. Kick-start the process by replacing one Really Bad lifestyle habit with a Really Good one – a cup of green tea instead of coffee is an excellent start. Put some effort in and substitute fruit in place of sweets, fresh veg in place of junk food.

Think fun when you think of exercise. Forget hiring a personal trainer or signing up for the gym, that's so last year! Source an exotic new way to get fit. We're talking yoga based aerobics in a funk 'n' grind atmosphere – looking hot doesn't have to be a bum deal! Use your imagination. Burlesque anyone? Pole dancing? Know your Foxtrot from your Slow-Shuffle and dazzle with your Quickstep. Engage in some full on physical fun with classes called Troubled Tums and Bubble Bums. Do it for the sake of your health *and* your self-esteem.  Sign up for lessons in self-defence salsa, samba, or just crank up the music and dance!

### 5 Top Tips
- Get the DVD if you can't get to a class
- Eat fresh food to increase your energy levels
- Perfect your body-nique – stripper-robics anyone?
- Generate energy/rhythm/endorphins and stretch yourself!
- Do One Good Thing everyday!

Get the infamous Dita Von Teese Look-at-Me posture by applying some poise enhancing exercise routines; throw in some power yoga or Pilates and a few basic rules to improve your body-nique. Study every aspect of your body language. Be smart about the signals your body is putting out there.

**Rule of thumb: Slouched body = bad self-image**

**Shoulders back, chest out, chin up = good self-image.**

- Use Naomi Campbell-esque posture to show that you're proud of your physique – whatever your size.

- Practice sitting and standing up straight, it doesn't matter if you're at work or in the privacy of your own home.

- Don't slump. It's not flattering and will add ten years to you! Throw that chest out and walk tall.

### *Stripmania!*

*Throw in some Wild Girl rules because nice gals don't always come first.* Get online and order Carmen Electra's *Advanced Aerobic Striptease* DVD if you want to give yourself or anyone you know some heart racing thrills and spills. Deck yourself out in lashings of eyeliner and red lipstick; pull on your leopard print bra, ripped Jack Daniels t-shirt and Guns N Roses headscarf! Practise getting comfortable with your body because once you've got your fancy-pants dance moves down pat, you're going to rehearse a slow, hot striptease! Don't worry, it's just in front of the mirror at this stage, you don't need to take it out into the real word – just yet! Once you start practicing, keep at it to get it down pat, you never know when you might need it ready to perform at the drop of a hat!

*Moral of the Story:* Get your gear off, smother yourself in a gorgeous creamy concoction and look in the mirror. Show your body some love and stop being afraid. No one's perfect, but there's nothing wrong with pretending!

# DAY 5

## *FASHION DIVA MODE*

Tune into the flirting channel to find new ways to refresh your wardrobe.

➢ Prepare a 'Just in Case' outfit ready to rock at a moments notice!

➢ Get all your favourite pieces and accessories out and experiment to see how many different new 'looks' you can create.

➢ Splash out on a tailor made garment, or invest in one piece of couture clothing that will make you look and feel better than you ever thought possible.

➢ Vamp it up with an outfit from another time. An animal print jacket coupled with a LBD, your hair curled up like a 40s movie star.

➢ Wear attention grabbing accessories – anything that will make you stand out from the pack and make it easy for someone to saunter over and say, "wow, I love your…." A geisha fan, a badge or fingerless gloves are a great start.

➢ Write down the `look' that you've always wanted to carry off but were never brave enough to try. The look that makes you feel ultra sexual and powerful. Now find an excuse to wear that outfit. All it takes is a bit of lateral thinking: if you can't find a theme night, you can create your own at-home themed party, either way, you get to dress up.

➢ Buy just one pair of shag-me-shoes!

# DAY 6
## BOOK A COSMETIC MAKE-OVER SESSION

*Step1.* Book yourself in to any department store for a cosmetic make-over. In most places the cost is redeemable for the purchase of one or two products. In other words, the makeover is free if you buy a lipstick and mascara. Do it before a big night out. Book with plenty of notice and be sure to prepare in advance by writing down details of the look so you can recreate the look later.

*Step 2.* Make the most of your hot new look by organising a photo shoot on the day. Figure out in advance what you will wear. Have several different changes of clothes, hairstyles and looks ready to go. Make an effort to totally restyle yourself. Think about who you will model yourself on and the style you will go for? Call a girly summit and get your Flirt Squad over to be part of the fun and then get ready for your close up!

*"It's fun to be a woman. It's fun to flirt and wear make-up and have boobs."*
-Eva Mendes

## *DAY 7*

## *THE GLAM QUIZ*

# FLIRT DIVA FUN AND GAMES

The way you carry yourself and the way you feel about your body says a lot about how you perform in the flirting department. It makes sense that of course we'll be better flirts if we're feeling gorgeous. What's your state of mind right now? Do you feel sexy, sultry and full of confidence? Or are you going through a hermit phase? Take this quiz to find out what your beauty and body loot say about you: your strong body suit and the areas you can work on. Discover more about your overall flirt style based on your beauty lifestyle.

1. ***Q. How's your beauty regime looking?***
   A. I'm afraid to say I've neglected myself recently.
   B. I wouldn't be seen dead without my slap, I stick to my regime religiously.
   C. I have a regime, but sometimes forget to stick to it.
   D. My regime goes up and down like a yo-yo. I'm always trying different products.
   E. I like the *theory* of a regime.

2. **Q. How's your body image these days? What can you do to improve it?**

   A. I don't have time to think about my body, my boss has me working all hours.

   B. I love my body – and so does everyone else!

   C. Well no one is perfect, but I don't spend much time worrying about it.

   D. I can't stand the way I look. I need cosmetic surgery!

   E. I'm not really happy with some aspects, but I know I can get into shape, if I put my mind to it.

3. **Q. What make-up do you always put on before leaving the house?**

   A. Just the basics: a little mascara and some lippy.

   B. The works! Foundation, blush, mascara, eyeliner and lippy.

   C. It depends where I'm going but usually just mascara, eyeliner and lippy.

   D. I always like to look polished, so I never leave the house without painting my face.

   E. I only wear make-up if I'm going somewhere special; otherwise it's just a bit of tinted moisturizer and lip balm.

4. **Q. Whose beauty style do you like the most?**

   A. Jennifer Aniston

   B. Gwen Stefani

   C. Kate Hudson

   D. Nicole Kidman

   E. Kate Moss

5. *Q. What's your signature beauty look?*

   A. My flawless complexion.

   B. Sexy come-hither eyes with glossy red lips.

   C. My hair. I like to mess it up: big and curly one day, sleek and straight the next.

   D. Pretty and polished make-up with super-shiny hair.

   E. My just-rolled-out-of-bed-with-a-lush-guy look.


6. *Q. What's the one beauty tool you can't live without?*

   A. Magnified mirror – ideal for checking out nasty blemishes.

   B. Eyelash curler.

   C. A hair iron.

   D. A hair curler.

   E. Hairbrush – I don't use much else!


7. *Q. When was the last time you went on a diet?*

   A. It's hard to stick to a diet when I'm constantly on the go.

   B. I always stick to a diet of fresh and organic food so I don't feel the need to try fad diets.

   C. I don't need to diet; I can pretty much eat whatever you want.

   D. Yesterday! I want to drop a few kilos ASAP.

   E. I'm always starting them, but aren't fussed enough to stick to them.

**8. Q. How do you feel about getting naked in front of a guy?**

    A. I'm only comfortable if I'm really drunk or the lights are out.

    B. Totally fine! If you've got it, flaunt it – I know I've got it!

    C. I'm not too worried about it.

    D. I don't get naked in front of a guy until I'm comfortable enough – I am a lady after all!

    E. I like my body, but I'm still a bit shy about showing it off.


**9. Q. What does your exercise routine include?**

    A. Getting up early to work out at the gym. Spinning works wonders when you're time poor.

    B. Does sex count? Other than that, I love my yoga.

    C. Strutting from boutique to boutique.

    D. I love running outdoors.

    E. Hitting the gym a few times a week.


**10. How much time do you spend pampering yourself?**

    A. Not much at all. After work and social commitments there's barely time for beauty treatments.

    B. I love indulging myself with massages and facials – I'm worth it!

    C. I treat myself to a facial every now and then, but my bank balance is more in favour of DIY.

    D. A fair bit: I like to look polished all the time so I'm always heading to the salon for waxing, shaping, tinting and pampering.

    E. Erm, I moisturise twice daily in the winter.

**Mostly As: You're a natural beauty.**

You take pride in the way you look, but busy work commitments make it hard for you to spend as much time on your appearance as you'd like to. You're comfortable with the way you look, but you'd love to be more confident about your body. Luckily for you, you look fabulous even with bare skin but when you do put the effort in, the results are striking. It may be hard to fit a little "you" time into your busy schedule, but try setting aside an hour a week to spend on DIY beauty maintenance.

**Mostly Bs: You're a sultry beauty.**

Congratulations! You are a great Flirt Diva in the making and you have a great attitude when it comes to the way you look. You're just as confident being stark naked as when you're dressed to the nines with a face full of perfectly-applied make-up. You know how to do yourself up to get a guy's attention – and how to keep it. Your confidence is a wonderful quality with instant 'in your face' appeal. Just make sure you don't spend *too* much time focusing on how you look.

**Mostly Cs: You're an experimental beauty.**

You're happy with the way you look. And you know which make-up and hair styles look best on you. This is a wonderful gift you have! You love experimenting with make-up tricks and techniques, and you're always working on cool, quirky ways to wear your hair – your trademark feature. Good on you for having a great relationship with your look and your body. While your confidence is not always apparent, you possess that subtle self-assurance that guys fall for over and over again.

**Mostly Ds: You're a feminine beauty.**

You're a girly girl and you're not afraid to show it. You love looking polished, and spend as much time as it takes perfecting your hair and make-up each morning so that you look positively gorgeous when you leave the house. While you're not one to follow crazy make-up trends, you're all for trying out different fad diets. You're a little unsure of your own beauty and find it hard to see yourself the way others see you. It's time to stop hiding and start flaunting your best assets.

**Mostly Es: You're a low maintenance beauty.**

You're not up with the latest trends in hair and make-up, but you don't need to be. You tend to look pretty good even when you've just rolled out of bed. You don't need to fuss around with eyeliner techniques and lipstick tricks and guys love that. You're so low maintenance! There's nothing that bugs them more than a girl who spends hours in front of the mirror! Just don't be afraid to surprise them every now and then by glamming yourself up. You'll be amazed at how sexy you will feel and how much more confident you'll be if you spend a little time on yourself. It's all about Inner Confidence. That means not letting your standards slip, or falling into the trap of being unprepared.

***Flirt Review: Finding your Signature Flirt Profile:***

Now that you've identified your beauty style, you should be getting a more vivid picture of your approach to femininity, and how it impacts on your ability to flirt. It goes without saying that if you look great, you feel great. And since you're getting a good sense of what works for you looks wise, you will make it your business to wow them every time you step out the door. In turn this will give you the confidence you need to flirt.

Under your Step 3 Flirt Review heading, write down any thoughts that come to mind about how your body image is working for you right now. Likewise if it's not working for you, what changes and improvements do you need to implement to get yourself looking and feeling the best you can? Flick back to Step 2's Celeb Flirt Quiz to see how compatible your beauty style is with your flirt style. Make a list of your body image priorities and pledge to action them!

# Congratulations you've completed your Step 4 missions!

## Step 4 Learning Outcomes

*Key points*

> ➤ Check your make-up in a naturally lit mirror before leaving the house.
> ➤ Do one thing everyday to make yourself feel more glam.
> ➤ Remember: it's impossible to see beauty though a sour expression!

*Checklist*

> ✓ Glowing health
> ✓ Lip-gloss & mascara (or course!)
> ✓ Lingerie by Agent Provocateur (recycle the bag so everyone knows you shop there!)
> ✓ A hat
> ✓ Queen of the F***** Universe T-Shirt

*Vamp Mantra:* *First impressions are everything and I'm not going to mess with mine!*

# Step 5 Chatarazzi: How to schmooze like a Flirt Diva!

## Week 5

In Step 5 we put the spotlight on the gamut of communication skills. We'll focus on the art of first-class conversation and of course, the power of listening, which is just as important. We'll look at different ways to sharpen your skills with ice-breakers, the art of accepting compliments and knowing the trade secrets behind making conversations more lively and fun.

*Key phrase*: *Communicate!*

*Challenge*: *Make others feel more at ease.*

*Goal:* *The ability to talk to anyone.*

*Result:* *Talking the talk!*

***Chapter 8. Read my lips not my hips***

As part of your Action Diva plan of attack, it's essential to have A-grade communication skills. It's not just what you say, but *how you say it.* If your chat skills aren't up to speed, you need to knuckle down and work on them – pronto. The ability to talk to anyone and have the knack of creating sparkling conversation should be your secret weapon when it comes to meeting someone special. Don't underestimate its importance.

In order to rate your communication skills, start by having a good, hard look at your Social Diva. How does she hold up in the harsh light of day? Maybe you think your mode of communication is full of beans, and maybe it is, in the smug 'n' comfy confines of your inner clique, but take you out of it and what happens? Do you dissolve? Turn into a quivering mess, one who doesn't cope very well making small talk with strangers at all? Or do you find you're such a nervous ball of energy that you can't shut-up, and no one else can get a single word in?

It's only natural that your conversations will seem awkward, disjointed or limited if you're out of practice. So, first things first. Stop operating from the back stalls and make a vow to get out of any hermit like behavioural patterns you might be trapped in. That means getting offline, getting out into the real world and letting yourself become momentarily intrigued by, oh I don't know, the sometimes forgotten art of a face-to-face conversation! It's called chatting – and it's a lifestyle tool. So let's turn you into a super communicator, someone who can tell a story in all its glory.

The secret of confident conversation stems from having the right attitude, which is really just knowing what you've got to offer, and putting it out there. Perhaps even more importantly though, it comes from *having a life* – which if you've been a goodliddle Flirt Diva and doing what you're told up until this point, yours should be brimming with good stuff! And once you've got something to talk about, it's the easiest thing in the world to convert into crackling sound-bites.

Entertaining a group and making them laugh can be heady, intoxicating fun, but not if your jokes are badly timed, poorly delivered and going down like a lead balloon. I know what that feels like! Laughter from good conversation lubricates the soul in the same way sex hormones lubricate the joints. And now that you're working on your hot new mindset, you should be thinking in terms of having a laugh. Your aim should be to generate a light, feathery pace from which you can tickle your flirt-mate's funny bone. It's all just bubble and froth really. And it's a lot of fun. Always remember, the buzz word isn't orgasm and the goal isn't sex – it's laughing! There's plenty of time for the heavy stuff later.

It's not just your social life that will benefit from your vamped up skills; other areas will flourish as well. How do you think the world's most successful entrepreneurs got to be that way? It was largely thanks to their ability to thrive on a big personality, spin a yarn and party like it's 1999! That's what's shot them into the business stratosphere. So don't ever underestimate the way your networking skills can help catapult your career, as well as your social standing.

The ability to express yourself confidently, whether it's one-on-one, in a group, or in front of a crowd, can have an astonishing effect on your social diary, your love life and the things you want out of life. That's where your imagination needs to kick in and do what ever it takes to top up your story-telling ability and apply it to everyday life. Your version of last night's events – about the home pizza delivery that went AWOL – should be as compelling as an Agatha Christie mystery. If it's not, summons in the professionals!

### Don't let your CSS – Chronic Shyness Syndrome – hold you back

The fear of public speaking has been rated as the all time number one phobia, with some introverts claiming, on record, that it is more feared than death. This is just nuts. It doesn't have to be that way. Now is the time to challenge all that old thinking and focus on overcoming the chat-clammies – often appearing in the form of stage fright, speech phobias or performance anxiety. All factors that can screw you over when it comes to Meeting New People.

The challenge is to electrify your storytelling skills – and you will, if you do just two things – 1) get a life and 2) practice! The most successful socialisers keep their conversations energetic and upbeat. They ask more questions and give longer, more thoughtful answers when they're asked something. They also understand the impact of offering personal details without being prompted. It has the effect of making the conversation seem more intimate. And they *always* use their flirt-mate's name – designed to make anyone feel oh-so special.

Help others relax by taking control and steering the conversation. Try it. You'll see that as soon as you put someone else in the spotlight and get them to talk about stuff they love, you'll always be sought out. It's just like being a world-class reporter and getting the big scoops. The guys who get those have a combination of two things: excellent communication skills designed to get to the heart of the matter, and charisma.

You'll find it the easiest thing in the world to crackle and pop with small talk once you've braved a performance in front of a roomful of strangers. Public speakers use lots of sneaky little tricks, and once again good old Jay-Z has some words of wisdom. *"Don't matter if it's 11 people or 11, 000." He says. "I just imagine them naked"* ♥. So hey, if it's going to help, knock yourself out!

Communicating with diva dexterity is one thing. But listening is quite another and newsflash – this can be the most powerful seduction tool you'll ever use. So, if you really want to hit those Flirt Diva highs, and focus the attention on your eyes, not your thighs, you need to master the art of *listening up!*

Any man or woman who can listen, without interrupting, is the sexiest thing alive. Truly! And really, are you ever listening? Or are you too busy looking at the label on his shirt, glancing at his shoes, eyeing up the brand on his watch, or the thickness of his wallet – because these are the things that really tell you who he is – not what he's saying? If that's the case, then you're barking up the wrong tree! Search his face and his conversation for clues, not his logos!

Right then, let's get to it. You can have a lot of fun with this but you will need to apply yourself. I can only say so much, the rest is up to you, you're the one who actually has to do it! You'll need to put in the effort to ramp up your new skills and once you do, you will find your confidence levels soar sky-high. Even more thrillingly, your new skills will help bring potential flirt-mates' out of *their* shell and ignite a real sense of getting along like a house on fire. These are the rewards you will reap as you learn to fire a frisky exchange along and master the art of flirt jargon.

So without any further ado, your Flirt Diva mission, should you choose accept it, is to make your flirt-mate feel like the World's Most Popular Man whilst convincing him that he has absolutely, one hundred percent, hit the jackpot with you. Lucky geezer!

---

♥ Jay-Z, Observer Music Monthly, 14 July, 2008

## Step 5

### 7-Day-Fill-Out-and-Keep-Flirt-Plan

*Day 1.* Prepare

*Day 2.* Sharpen Up

*Day 3.* Yes, but what do I say?

*Day 4.* Question Time

*Day 5.* Accept that Compliment, Damn You!

*Day 6.* Becoming an Observational Super Power

*Day 7.* Listen Up!

# *DAY 1*

# *PREPARE*

Prepare your best stories and gags by writing them down and committing them to memory. That way they will always be ready to roll out with a seconds notice, and you won't have that experience of "freezing" half way through a story when you realise you've forgotten some crucial detail, or worse, the punch line. And believe me, it happens. My friends' don't call me "goldfish" for nothing.

Likewise, think about where you are going before you head out. Think about the people you will meet and the things you will have in common – whether that's music, cocktails, food or pool. Spend ten minutes mentally rehearsing ice-breakers and conversation boosters so you don't break into a cold sweat if someone approaches you. Alternatively if you feel up to making an approach, or simply prompting someone to get them talking back to you, you'll have some cracking ice-breakers which will make the approach seem infinitely less terrifying!

*"I'm a tryer. I've done the best with my talent that I can."*

- J.K Rowling, when asked to describe herself.

# DAY 2

## RESEARCH COMMUNICATION SKILLS

There is a whole world of fun things to do that will help in your pursuit of becoming a communicator extraordinaire. Take your pick. There's every sort of confidence booster imaginable, all designed to dramatically improve your ability to click and connect.

Consider acting lessons, stand up comedy classes, public speaking, or even teaching lessons. Enrol for a story-telling session or singing lessons. Look into courses and online workshops. This Flirt Diva has done them all. They're brilliant. If none of those are available, download online courses or read a book on the subject. There are some great ones about. I recommend *How to Talk to Anyone* by Leil Lowndes.

---

**He'll never forget the night he met you.** You sashayed into that bar, and even though you weren't the best looking babe in the room, you had an aura and you caught his eye. It's not because you were wearing your frontless, backless get up, but because you moved with confidence and poise, always a magnet for the boys. You looked up, caught his eye and showered him with a slow, sexy smile. He recognized it as the Green Light and beamed back it right back. You rewarded him with your biggest *fancy-a-flirt-smirk* and waved him over; within minutes he'd dragged himself away from his mates and was snaking his way towards you. Straight away he could tell there was something special going on with you, a quality he hadn't seen in many girls. And you knew it too. You were on fire, charming, chatty, and hilarious, but you stood aside to let him take the floor. Many cheeky grins and great flirting trademarks later, he passes you his card, raises his brow and smilingly asks for your number. You flip the card over, scribble it down and toss it back. He doesn't bother about his usual three-day rule. He calls you the next day. *This is the stuff that will happen if you start practicing now!*

---

## DAY 3
## YES, BUT WHAT DO I SAY?

Banter will fizzle not sizzle if it's left for too long, so you need to be out there practicing regularly. You can practice on anyone, anywhere, anytime. Ditch your play-it-cool mantra and start sparking up conversations from scratch. Ease your way in by practicing on little old ladies – seriously! They love to have a chat and they don't get that many people to talk to, so you'll be performing a random act of kindness as well! Find your own technique to jump-start conversations. Hit upon some common ground and just go for it. It doesn't matter where you are. Just make the most of every opportunity.

Once you've got your ice-breakers under control, it will be easy to get things warmed up and crackling along in no time. Anything that starts with *"Hello, I don't think I've ever had a full lesbian experience, but…"* is guaranteed to get his interest. (Just for the record I don't actually recommend this tactic!) Start a low-fi chat while you're standing around and use whatever props are there. So say there's a pool table, you can start off with a chat about the game and move onto the crowd, the music, the venue, the location, the DJ, the price of drinks – anything at all really! If he's not into it – so what? Walk away! It's not like you asked him to father your child. And who knows, maybe he's just a sad bastard. Emotional detachment, remember? It's his loss but your gain because it's proof that you're getting on top of managing the conversational heebie-jeebies.

If on the other hand he's receptive and it's all going swimmingly, revert back to the default position – question time! Ask where he got his natty shoes, what music he likes, what sport he's into and what he does in his spare time. From there it's a simple leap to bringing out his fun side.

That can mean getting in touch with *his* inner child by cheering him on, telling silly gags and prompting *his* stories by playfully reminding him of the best day of his life – simply by asking about it. Shower him with your most orgasmic smile and clasp his hand with both of yours. Look him in the eye and compliment him on his smile, his shirt, his…whatever!

And relax…

Now imagine you're standing at the bar waiting to order when a hot dude with a big tempting grin props up *right next to you.* With a hip thrust and a hair flick that would put Shakira to shame, you volley that grin right back at him. *"I guess I should introduce myself,"* you say, fluttering your lashes, swaying your hips, flipping and tucking your hair. Then throw in something light and silly to fit the situation:

*"I'm taking a poll for the bar, which do you prefer?*

" Beer or cider?"

" Footy or cricket?"

" Cats or dogs?"

You get your drinks and *of course,* he's not going anywhere, he's hanging around for a chat. So far so fabulous. Well done you!

### Yes, but what do I say?

And then, it happens, after a promising start, all high energy and seductive smiles, you find you've got nothing to say! So what do you do? Well there's no black and white formula, but you'll be fine if you start by making the most of the environment – you have that in common.

- I love this band! You seen them before? What do you think?
- I'm not a smoker, but I feel sorry for anyone who has to stand outside and freeze their butts off…how about you?

- I had a massive night last night and danced all night. What did you do?

Next, whip out a little conversational nugget that you prepared earlier – even better if it's a wee bit embarrassing. I'll have you know it's been scientifically proven that anyone who can have a laugh at their own expense is irristable. It's endearing and shows a hint of vulnerability – that makes it crucial to seduction. So you're not perfect? Who would've known? Right then, off you go…

***Avoid the case of: "Too much, too soon!" Flirt Divas don't tell all their secrets!***

*Have a laugh at your own expense, but don't go overboard. He doesn't have to know:*

- What happened behind the shelter sheds That Day.
- That you're paranoid, impatient and self-conscious.
- You hate your ingrown bikini hairs.
- And don't see why you should have a Brazilian wax every freakin' month!

- 

*Remember the Vamp Mantra: Too much information!*

Avoid gossip, gobbledygook and girly stuff – anything that will scare him off.

*Newsflash: Men are terrified of neurotic women. Correction. We all are!*

175

A lifetime of oestrogen can make you want to start bitching and whining about your boss or something equally dull, but try to refrain. Your flirt-mate doesn't need to see your natural pessimism – just yet!

### *Fancyadrinkthen?*

Things are going well, and you're feeling both bolshy and generous, so you offer to buy the next drink – well, why not?

**What you could say with a big grin is:**

- *You look thirsty and I'm going to the bar. Shall I bring you back a drink?*
- *You look like you could do with a Long Tall Glass of something fabulous. Fancy it?*

*And now you've given him his cue to but the next round. You're just prompting him remember – leading by example. If he doesn't take the hint, you can either give him another hint, or walk away.*

### Fancyadancethen?

**Example #1**: So you've moved in nice and close and found flirty excuses to touch his arm, his shoulder, his hand. You're toying with him now, *you Flirt Diva you,* and it's all going very smoothly. You like this guy, you've got a good feeling about him, and you want him to come out with you afterwards. So instead of making it sound like a life or death situation, keep the mood nice and light and use a technique that's called "presuming the sale".

**What you should say is:**

*"I'm thinking about bedroom accessories and how good you would look as one."* I'm kidding!

**What you should really say is:**

*"So we're all hitting a club soon. You'll be coming out with us yeah?"*

Accompanied by a big saucy grin. Works like a dream. Of course it's cocky, but, Flirt Diva, that's the point!

What you should **not** say is in a state of heightened anxiety is:

*"My friends are leaving in 10 minutes. We're going to a club. I need to tell them RIGHT NOW if I'm leaving with them. So, do you want to come or what?"*

**Example #2**: Let's say you've wound up at the same party; you give him your biggest smile and let your shoulder brush against his as you throw out a Flirt Diva lifeline accessorised by a very cheeky grin:

*I hope you know I'm planning on dancing my head off tonight – with you!"*

That'll do the trick. It's sexy, but not too OTT and it gives him the go-ahead to make the next move. If not, wait a suitable amount of time before you tell him, 'OMG'I-love-this-song!', grab his hand and hit the dance-floor.

*What do I do when his friend comes over?*

Aha! A golden opportunity to flash the Secret Smile. And, if you're feeling really frisky, bobble that eyebrow girlfriend! Establish that cosy sense of intimacy between the pair of you by acting like old mates. There's no better way to make people comfortable.

*Best not to try:*

- Taking the piss out of his hairdo (to his mate)
- Telling the mate, "he's 'hot!"
- Going all shy and quiet
- Telling his mate to take a hike so you can have him all to yourself

- Turning into Miss Potty mouth
- Asking his views on men waxing their privates

**Try strengthening the bond by talking about <u>him</u> to his mate:**
*"So your friend here was just telling me that a little old lady fainted on the train and he got her to safety." You look at him and beam a look of respect and swoon, "my hero!"*

### *Next on the schedule – Melting Man Moments*

You need an attitude that doesn't flip at the sight of a hot guy, so run through this list and add in *your own experiences and suggestions about what to say…*.

Best approach to use on a stranger
Example: *Smile and say "love your shirt. I bought one just like it for my brother recently."*
… … … … … … … … … … … … … … … … … … … … … … … … … … … … … …
Best way to drive a conversation?
Example: *So you do martial arts? Wow! How did you get into it?*
…………………………………………………………………………………..

Best line you've ever used:
Example: *Cor, are you in a famous band then?*
…………………………………………………………………………………
Best way to signal interest during the conversation:
Example: *Smile, use strong eye contact and keep prompting with questions*
…………………………………………………………………………………

*If all the above goes swimmingly and you want to add some spice to the conversation you could ask if he's tried:*

a) Phone sex?

b) Orgasm gel?

c) Any good aphrodisiacs lately?


*Or you could tell him the one about* the Orgasm Squad who arrested two over zealous Flirt Divas for illegal consumption of orgasms. Orgasm police say it came after an investigation into a ring of raging oversexed women which may result in several more arrests. Three of the suspects have pleaded guilty and agreed to attend 'orgasm rehab'. Further arrests for Flirt Diva offenders of the Permanently Horny Syndrome (PHS), which increases blood flow to the sex organs and enforces up to 200 orgasms a day, are likely to be made.

*That should get his interest!*

# DAY 4
## QUESTION TIME

OK, folks, it's question time. So get ready to ask away. And don't be shy, everyone loves being asked questions, I'm talking personally of course! In fact, the more questions, the better. It shows you're interested and you want to know more. It's actually very flattering. Listen closely to what someone's saying to help generate a line of friendly questioning – not an interrogation!

So, instead of asking the rather mundane: "How was your day?" which can get a mumbled jumbled response, especially if someone's had the day from hell, ask specific questions. Use any ammo you've gathered from snippets about anything at all that's going on in their lives. Perhaps they've recently changed jobs or careers. Ask how they're coping with the "change", rather than the bog standard, "How's work?"

I remember when I made the terrifying leap from the 9-5 job into a freelance career, and was experiencing a really tough time, how I wished my friends had asked the big questions, rather than assuming it was all going fine, because it wasn't!

### What if your flirt-mate answers everything with a 'Yes' and 'No' answer?

So you've given him a wink and a smile and engaged in a bit of chit chat; he's laughing and loving your company, so you leave it there in a, *"that'll do you for starters big boy"* kind of way. He's left wide-eyed and mesmerised. You come back later and you're two volleys in, but you're not getting any response beyond "yes" or "no" answers. If that's the case then either he's a monosyllabic deadbeat, or you're asking questions *the wrong*

180

*way*. The right way is to ask open-ended questions which invite more than a basic "yes" or "no" answer. So instead of:

*"Seen any good movies lately?"*

Try:

*"I've always wanted to play Lara Croft in Tomb Raider. Who's your superhero?*

Instead of:

*"Been on any good holidays lately?"*

Try:

*"I loved Ireland when I went there last year. I discovered Guinness and drank enough to sink a pirate ship. Where would you go back to visit, if you could go anywhere?"*

**Generally we make statements that encourage one word responses:**

*"Great party huh?"*

And then you're left wondering what on earth to say when you get an answer like:

*"Yep!"*

Yet if you tried:

*"Great party. How do you know our hostess?"*

And the answer is:

*"Steve and I went to high-school together."*

Jackpot! Now you've got a wealth of material to mine which makes it easier to continue the questions loosely based around the topic:

*Where did you grow up? Why did you move? What do you like best about living in the new place?*

This way you're prompting answers which can glide down another intriguing path as you establish the things you have in common. Stay in sleuth mode and find clues to keep things crackling along. You'll soon find yourself enjoying the sensation of driving this show and watching it fork off here and there. This truly is the holy grail of brilliant banter.

*Golden Rule: Keep things in perspective: it's a social networking exercise not a boyfriend-seeking mission! And hey, even if you don't like the guy, he might have a friend you fancy - so be nice!*

### *Filler questions to keep things firing along:*

- First record or CD you bought?

- Last CD you bought?

- Where in the world would you most like to be?

- Luxury item on a desert island?

- Three words your best mate would use to describe you?

- How far would you go on a first date? NO just joking, NEVER ask this!

### *Use the "What's your favourite..?" openers to fall back on:*

These are brilliant because you can literally ask about anything: movie, band, concert city, country, cuisine, bar, club, restaurant, sport, hobby, experience, animal, holiday, adventure...you get the picture!

*Or try the "tell me about ..." approach*

Your best ever day

Your craziest day

Your fantasy holiday

*Or use any of the What, Where, Who questions to get things rolling*

- Where did you find..?
- Who taught you to..?
- Where did you learn to..?
- What do you love about..?
- What do you like about...?
- What do you think about...?

*Have plenty of random questions at the ready:*

- Which 3 superstars would you invite to your birthday bash?
- Who would play your leading man in a movie about your life?
- What's your best party trick?
- If you could live anywhere in the world where would it be?
- What's your best joke?
- Are you a jocks or boxers man? *Or maybe not!*

*Try to use "Tag" questions. It's fine to talk about yourself as long as you include your flirt-mate! Stick to subjects that are relevant and you'll find your rhythm soon enough:*

- *I'm planning a trip away for the Bank Holiday weekend. What about you – any plans to go away?*
- *This is my first time at this bar. How about you, been here before?*
- *I haven't tried Thai before this, but I love it! What do you think of it?*

*Now you try. Write down 3 of your best questions/ice-breakers…*

1.
2.
3.

### Best way to signal that you'd like to know more

If you're feeling like a courageous Flirt Diva, why not suggest that you continue this shindig another time? It's easy if your flirt-mate is asking loads of animated questions in response to an interest of yours, just come right out and say it: *"If you're really interested we could meet up later and I could show you."*

### Or if you're a very brave Flirt Diva in the making, try:

*"Hey, I'm up for catching up same time next week if you're about?"*
If he's mentioned his penchant for French food, a passion you just happen to share, all you need to follow with is:
*"I'm always up for trying new places. Why don't we hook up and try one? How about same time next week?"*
Then, whip out your phone, ask for his number, and call it right then and there. Voila, now he's got your number as well! It's brazen but foolproof. If he still doesn't get it, you know the drill. Step away from the man!

➤ And now, if you're feeling really, really brave, take your new skills out and road test them on a stranger, (just be aware of stranger danger rules and don't do anything silly, just keep it light and fun). You can either give someone a random compliment, or start a mini conversation by incorporating your environment and the props around you.

➤ Always prepare ahead for what you will say and who you might encounter along the way. Think about the ways you will strike up a conversation. Organize your ice-breakers, put on your observational super-power hat and make sure you have plenty of generic compliments up your sleeve!

*Flirt Alert: Don't be a flirting snob, flirt with anyone and everyone.* Exercise a random act of kindness – just march right up to someone who looks frazzled, give them your best smile and hit them with your best compliment.

# DAY 5

## ACCEPT THAT COMPLIMENT DAMN YOU!

Giving compliments are crucial in that it really does have a magical effect on almost anyone – so long as they're genuine of course! But did you know that accepting compliments is just as much of an art?

*When someone gives you a compliment you should not:*

- Tell them they must be blind.
- Ask them what their problem is.
- Say can't we just cut to the chase already?
- Bore them with a lengthy explanation.
- Scowl and say, "Yeah right!"

*Instead you should try:*

- It's my favourite as well! I love it because…
- Thank you. I got it while I was travelling in….
- Thank you!

*Now you say it. Out loud!*

Now practice the art of *giving* a compliment. Put your thinking cap on and get your head around the mind-boggling array of compliments you can come up with in almost any situation.

## Food for thought:

- You remind me of that movie star from…
- You've got film star hair.
- You look like that rock star – whathisname?
- I noticed you when you walked in.
- You've got a real presence.
- I like the way you think!
- The world needs more people like you.
- I feel like I've known you forever!
- You remind me of a *really* close friend.

## Now list your Top Three

1.

2.

3.

## The Adios Compliment:

Reserved for Vamps in Training, the Adios compliment allows you to dart up to someone and dash off before they have a chance to reply. The benefits are twofold. First you get to make someone's day with a cool compliment (and that's always nice) and secondly, you don't run any risk of rejection. It's brilliant! It's also a nice way to *ease* into the land of compliments.

Select your target and focus in on that individual thing that's jumping out. Maybe it's a scarf, a pair of shiny shoes, a belt or bulging biceps. It could be anything. Everyone's got something worth complimenting; you'll know what you're looking for. And then, as you wander by, just mosey on up with a smile and say:

*"Hey, I just had to let you know that shirt looks FAB on you!"*

Flash that smile again, and shimmy away. A little something for him to think about later, hmmm?

**Throw him a compliment:**
- Nice shirt, wheredidya geddit?
- Great jacket
- Cool shoes!
- Nice tattoo
- Love the hat!

*Top Tip: Give someone, anyone a compliment. Who cares if you don't know them? It will make them feel fantastic.*

*After all these years of silence and abstinence, if I only remembered that I only had to smiled, I'd have done it sooner.*

- Anon.

# DAY 6
## BECOME AN OBSERVATIONAL SUPER POWER

Make a conscious decision to remember names. It's pretty basic stuff, but surprisingly few people actually *do it*. Use this trick to help you link names and faces. Once you've been introduced to someone, just stop for a second, look at them and take the time to absorb their name. Then, think of someone else you know with the same name, visualise them and link the two names together, saying it three times over to yourself. Simple! If you don't know anyone with the same name, use an object or a rhyme to help you remember. So if someone's name is Hailey, you might think about Hailey's Comet. Or Shawn might become lawn or fawn. Be as silly as you like, so long as it's memorable, who cares?

Use this strategy to apply for memorising facts and information as well, simply by using funny images as mental reminders. It's easy once you get into the habit. Take pride in your ability to remember names, faces and facts, and you'll stand out in the crowd because you'll be the only one who's bothered!

### Observational Super Power

If you want to be an observational super power (and who doesn't?) you've got to start focusing. That means really looking at someone when you're having a big old chat-fest. Start with their physical assets. What colour eyes do they have? What type of complexion? What style of hair and what skin type? Look closely at the whites of their eyes, their pupils, the condition of their hair, the texture of their skin. Then study their clothes. Pay attention to their overall style, the fabrics they're wearing, and their accessories. Try to summarise what their clothes say about them? See if you can come away

189

with a snapshot description worthy of the world's best photo journalist.

*Test your powers of observation by trying the following game with a friend*
Ask a trusted friend to blindfold you. (add some fluffy handcuffs if you like!) Next have them grill you for specific details about their appearance. Describe the shoes they're wearing; the colour and texture of their shirt. Are they wearing a belt? A watch? A ring? Or any other accessories? Describe anything else you've noticed about them. Take the blindfold off to see how effective your super powers are.

*Top Tip: Memorise names to be the life of the party.*

*And when you get home write up a little Charm School Card with the description and details of those you met tonight, so that if and when you bump into them again, you're not left floundering.*

♥           ♥           ♥

# DAY 7
## LISTEN UP!

Face it, almost everyone loves to talk about – you guessed it – themselves! So let them. Treat your best mate to a mock game of the TV show *This Is Your Life* down at your local pub. Give them the floor; give them the thrill of *An Evening Devoted to Them*. Let them walk away thinking you're the conversationalist of the century because *they had the time of their life.* You'll find that once you get into the habit of shining the spotlight on anyone and everyone, you'll soon be the real star of the show. The results will be addictive – and once you get a taste of the gratitude, you'll want more.

The only way to become a good listener is – you guessed it – with practice. So start now! Get into the habit of starting conversations with a smile and killer eye-contact, ask questions, listen carefully to the answers and cruise assertively down that path. Learn to recognize conversational clues and signposts, and pick up on them. Make it your flirting mandate to get a stranger or someone special to open up about themselves – or just get Anthony from accounts to tell you all about his weekend for god's sake. By listening closely for the clues, you will start to sprinkle stardust throughout your small talk and turn it into something unforgettable.

*"There are a lot of big egos in this business. When people act like divas, I smile at them, and let them talk – it clearly makes them happy. You can come away with great quotes if you listen."*
– Estelle

191

*Ok, Supergirl, quick spot-check to see how you're progressing so far...*

*Tick any of the following **if** they apply:*

1. *Have you been studying your female role models?*
2. *Signed up for any new challenges?*
3. *Done anything out of your comfort zone?*
4. *Gone out with platonic male friends to practise flirting?*
5. *Done any "couple watching"*
6. *Made any good eye contact with the opposite sex?*
7. *Flirted with anyone new?*

**If you ticked mainly No's, but you're serious about wanting the full Flirt Diva experience, you will need to go back and refocus on your weak areas.**

**If you ticked Yes! More than 4 times, you're on track. Yay you!**

## *Flirt Review: Finding your Signature Flirt Profile:*

Now that you've worked through the all important communication chapter, you should be getting a sense of how you can kick butt socially with the simple addition of some shiny new chat skills.

Make your Step 5 heading and write down any further suggestions about how you can continue to improve up your social confidence. What areas need to advance, and what actions will you take to become the ultimate communication diva?

While you're doing this, consider the day-to-day ways your new communication skills can impact on your life. For example, describe a fantasy situation – say you were to unexpectedly bump into 'him' the one and only McDreamy – what would you say and how would you handle yourself? Write down the imaginary scenario now! That way, if and when it does happen, you'll be prepared!

# Congratulations, you have completed your Step 5 missions!

## Step 5 Learning Outcomes

*Key points:*

> ➤ Be proud of who you are and what you stand for.

> ➤ Don't be afraid to be animated – you're here to entertain.

> ➤ Don't hold back.

*Checklist*:

✓ A swagger of stories and jokes

✓ A fearless approach to conversation

*Vamp Mantra*: *Interested equals interesting!*

# Step 6. Vamparazzi: How to sizzle like a Flirt Diva

*Week 6*

Here's where we bring it altogether. Step 6 is devoted to the full repertoire of flirting gestures. Here you'll find the complete A-Z of – what to do! All the signals and signs – yours, his, everybody's! You'll find ways to decode the language – as in "read" him and lots of other tricks and tips. Finally, you will complete the final phase of building your own personal signature style. Sound good?

*Key phrase:* *Awareness.*

*Challenge: Practice daily!*

*Goal: Find your signature style.*

*Result: Hitting your stride.*

### Chapter 9. Putting it all together to become a killer flirt

So here we are in the final phase of your flirting odyssey. Wahay! By now you should getting the hang of this flirting shtick and feeling the buzz of being psyched up. You're feeling empowered, you're feeling alive – honey you're on fire!

This is the time you channel *all your diva dexterity* to get a result, and convert your energy into getting out there and ultimately, *getting it on.* It's all about spinning the chase and turning it into the cha-cha-charm dance. That means playing it smart, paying attention and laying it on the line. You're conquering those L-plate nerves and advancing to flirting superstardom. Well done you. This is a celebration of you; a tribute to you. And deservedly so, because you little lady, are a mighty fine catch! That's the message. You don't need to say it. But you sure as hell need to think it. Get this in the bag and it will add up to a big fat A-plus in flirting. *Pantomime applause please!*

As you wave goodbye to the insecurities, doubts, fears and all those non-diva like traits that held you back previously; and ditch those distracting thoughts about marriage, mortgage and maternity dresses, all the M words – at least for now – you will start to feel great, which will have a domino effect and make others feel great as well.

So it's time to hit some home runs, whether that's getting loved up, trialling some flirtatious boy energy, or becoming more of a social butterfly than you ever dreamed possible. You're clued up to the eyeballs with the theory. You know what to say. Now you just need to know what to *do!* So what better time than to get started on the tactical stuff? Like the ability to mesmerise and hold anyone totally in your power. This is dead easy. It's the fun part! This is where the thrills and spills kick in as you step up to the plate to try your hand at your new skills. So here it is, the moment you've been waiting for - we've arrived at the engine room, the Central Nerve system. So deep breath, shoulders back, chin up, tummy in and smile. You want va va voom? We'll give you va va voom baby!

### Nothing says "let's get it on!" like a game of the "touchy feelies"

A true flirting pow-wow has the same ability to take your breath away and make you feel all woozy and light-headed. It's mystical and magical – but unlike a hallucinogenic – it doesn't screw with your health! Think swoon inducing passion, romance chemistry. *Zing. Wow. Kapow.* Watch Audrey Hepburn's Holly Golightly lean in to kiss the salesman in *Breakfast at Tiffany's* to get her wicked way. See how she shimmies in nice and close and gives an adorable little shoulder shrug while she murmurs breathlessly into her lover's ear. Ultimately these are the slivers of gold that blend together to help you find your flirting feet. And you will find your rhythm, but like anything worthwhile, it requires commitment, which judging by your application so far, you've got in droves!

In an ideal world you will be able to monitor how you are coming across right at that moment when you ignite your inner temptress and unleash the perfect "10" hair-flick. So long as you practice at home in front of the mirror first, and yes, you may feel like a git, but don't let that stop you!

The crucial thing – and we'll go through this in more detail in the challenges –is *not to let your flirt-mate miss the cues and signals* and remember, *if you are too subtle*, he will almost definitely miss them. So be direct, but keep it all under control. Flutter your lashes by all means, but blink too hard and for too long and he'll just think you've got something lodged in your eye. You're going for flirt queen, not epileptic queen!

We'll look at the strategy of volume and repetition – a sure fire approach as you dish out your top-of-the-line-no-poncy bollocks moves. Thrust out all those seriously sexy signs that tell him you're keen, and just keep playing your hand until you see that flicker of recognition cross his face. Bang him over the head with your jostling, jiggling, jiving and jazzin' and then relax and wait for the signs to come hurtling back. And if he misses it, or chooses to ignore it, then he's a lame duck and you're out of luck. And yes, things can misfire. If that happens and he's not reciprocating (or worse still looking alarmed) – you can easily make out that you were just mucking around as mates. The Flirt Diva is nothing if not mischievous.

Happily there are no hard and fast rules when it comes to flirting, in spite of what the textbooks tell you. So don't worry about getting too bogged down with technical detail. Just be confident that you're broadcasting your message as clearly as possible and trust that nature will do the rest. The bonus is that flirting can't be one-sided. Well actually it can, but it's a bitch to keep flirting when you're doing it on your lonesome! And if your flirt-mate's not flirting back, you'll know about it soon enough! You may step on a few toes, just like dancing, but so what? You'll become more skilled over time. And even if you do stumble a bit, who cares? Just get back out there.

And that, my smitten kittens, is the language of the true flirt. It's just a game, and it's meant to be fun. A hotbed of lusty body contact, a playful push and pull of limber limbs, shameless grins, wandering thighs and lingering eyes. It's powerful but understated, sexual but sensual, sassy but sultry.

Just to recap, don't be pinning all your hopes on this chance meeting resulting in the love of a lifetime – that's just jumping the gun. This is the time to loosen up, concentrate on the banter, have a laugh and get those points ticking on the flirt-o-meter!

### *Flirt Alert – mischief suggests unpredictability in the bedroom*

So now ladies, prepare to take the floor as the queen of your own flirt-show; a place where you are limited only by your romantic imagination. Settle in at Flirt Diva Central and get ready for a bit of fluff 'n' fun as we cross-examine the mystifying smorgasbord of flirting signals, codes and gestures.

And fear not, I've taken into account that it's early days and you may be still feeling a little awkward, but I know you're up for the challenge. It just takes practice and repetition. *Practice and Repetition. Practice and Repetition.*

First we're going to find your "on" switch. So rather than stepping out and basking in your existing meat-and-two-veg flirt repertoire – the blink-and-you-miss-it-hair-flick, stingy lip-lick and glazed-eyed sex-slave-stare – because that's never going to bring that bad boy home – we're going to expand your range. We'll get those lash-aerobics working overtime and incorporate dozens of fancy new moves which will blow his tiny little mind.

To begin with, you'll need to get the Flirt Squad around quick smart so you can practise in the privacy of your own home; *before* you take your fancy schmancy moves out on the town and road-test them in front of your new fanclub. We don't want you getting banned from anywhere after any incidents involving sexual harassment!

So big breath now, there's a lot to get through, but it's all good stuff. Above all it's empowering in that supersonic *I'm Every Woman* way. You're no longer Miss Wing It. You know how to avoid Mr Yeah Right! and you're able to spot a Red Flag danger man at one hundred paces. Excellent! Now let's try out a few flirting staples, like how to stand . . .

*mmmm* a little closer. Smile in that…*ahhhh* way. Make excuses to…*ooooh-er* graze his shoulder.

OK, so you're out. You're flirting. You're fabulous. You're brushing his arm with every hilarious punch line, extending your eye contact, smouldering and moving in closer with every breathless sentence. You're asking open ended questions (if he was a super-hero who would he be?) and the conversation is flowing like the most divine wine. But wait, are you paying attention to the signals he's sending back? Because if you're not, you're only having half the fun.

When it comes to duo-flirting, your power-hand lies with a technique known as *multi-tasking* and hey, you're a woman, you're good at that! So rather than just dishing out the signals, you've got to watch for them to come flowing back in. Rule of thumb, when two of you are involved in the flirting-rumba, one of you will have the upper hand. That person will be the big cheese, the mistress of ceremonies, the dominating flirt. They will lead and set the mandate. If things are going exceptionally well, the roles can reverse half way through and your flirt-mate will pick up the slack – this is a truly great sign. But at the end of the day it's a power game and if you start it, you've got to finish it. It's up to you to close the deal. Dem's da rules.

### So, how do you know when he's flirting back?

In a perfect world, your flirt-mate would respond by demonstrating the classic "I'm into you" moves. If he's switched on enough that is. Here's what he'd do: he'd twist his torso around so he's facing you; point his feet towards you; look at you adoringly for just a moment to long; ogle your lips, and he'd probably also look a little bewildered, but in a good way! Remember he's not the expert at this stuff, you are!  Just keep an eagle eye

201

on his signals, but be patient. It can take a while before you're good enough to decipher the code, especially when you're busy beaming out your own message! It can seem tricky at first, but soon it will be as easy as riding a rickshaw.

Keep in mind there are no foolproof rules and nothing is set in stone; so if he inadvertently twists his body *away* while you're attempting to flirt, you simply can't assume it's not working or that he's not interested – at least not until you've seen the same negative signs repeated a few times over – then you can take the hint. A lot of what we say and do is instinctual, so to begin with, it's just a matter of becoming more attuned to that process. If it gets to the point where he's not hanging on to your every word, or even pretending to be enthralled by your goddess like presence, you can be pretty sure, he's just not that into you (unless he's super shy in which case you can throw him a goddamn bone).

Let me share a little Flirt Diva story with you. This was back in the day when I had a mad crush on the `Speed-Freak' – otherwise known as my erm, university lecturer! We were having our end of term party and I'd been planning and scheming for weeks, little minx that I was. I'd planned my outfit in excruciating detail, certain that this was the night he would fall madly, badly in love with me.

It started off promisingly enough. The two of us greeted each other with rapturous smiles and sat cross-legged on the floor sharing a cider listening to *Smashing Pumpkins*. And then, as I was halfway through a story (that I clearly thought was fascinating), he ever so casually yawned and did a purposeful sweep of his watch. I nearly died! I totally dropped the ball after that. I couldn't imagine why I'd want to stay and talk with someone when the only effect I was having seemed to be making them think about where else they could be! It wasn't long afterwards that I found out he had a live-in girlfriend. Oops. Well at least I didn't ignore the signals, and in hindsight, I may have saved myself a lot of pain in the long-term.

The message is DO read the signs. DON'T ignore them. And don't badger someone who isn't responding positively; or keep pushing them to go out with you if they're reticent from the beginning. You might get them in the short term – but you'll never keep them – and that's a promise. Added to that, they'll always have the upper hand simply because you like them more than they like you.

### So what's all this about chasing men then?

By now you would agree that to attract a man successfully, just your average, attractive cheeky chappie, you need to get your head out of the comfort cone and into the flirting zone. You're clear that like anything else in the world you aspire to, you need to push yourself and be willing to face the good with the bad. Now is absolutely the right time to get busy and find someone nice and low-fi to practice on. Once you start spending time around males in general, you'll find the conversational patter comes more naturally, so you really need to hop to it. If you've been practicing while you're out and about, you will be feeling ready to strike like a coiled snake the second you see someone who looks decent enough and of course, not too threatening!

You'll know you're doing it right if the seductive scent of danger fills your nostrils. Because that's fear, and it's healthy. It's an inner barometer that tells us we're alive. That's what propels us along when we charge out to the forefront of life with reckless excitement, electrifying potential flirt-mates all across the land, making us feel like goddamn warriors. Knowledge is power and right now you are getting powered up to the eyeballs. And that's a big bonus when it comes to overcoming fear.

Your ego smells fear and will try like hell to trip you up. Do whatever you need to stay calm and focused. So what if you need a dirty martini to loosen up – when was that ever a problem?

Just try not to get too carried away. Keep things low risk by lowering the stakes. Make it easy on yourself. You should be revelling in the random hilarity of it all. Learn to relax and enjoy it. That's the point after all, it should be fun. Totally mentalist fun. Especially when you stretch those boundaries as far as you can – without going over the edge of course. Take the pressure off by getting out there to practice when it *doesn't* count – like with someone who won't make you break out in a nervous rash! Rather than leaving everything to the Omigod! moment you stumble across the man of your fantasies. And having to face up to your insecurities, or worse still, his!

### And approach…

Sometimes you just wish for that fantasy moment, where you lock eyes with a dreamy guy and he swoops you up in his arms and take the lead right from the word go. But, it doesn't always happen that way does it? That's why I want to talk about the big difference between chasing someone – and being open about the fact you like them.

For the record, I don't believe in chasing anyone. It smacks of desperation. But no-one's saying that the act of making a simple approach is chasing. Nor are they saying you have to broadcast it with a post-it note on your forehead. That's just not cool. Having said that, I also know that some of the best men on the planet are totally clueless. And lord knows, they need a nudge. So if you've got the chutzpah to wander over and say "hey!" you could be the one walking away saying, "result!"

Picture the scene. There you are and there he is. Preppy boy, square-jawed martini-drinking suit, pretty-boy gangster, slick hip-hopper or floppy haired intellectual. Whatever you fancy – he's it. He's sauntered over to the bar to order a pint. He looks around, he sees you and – shock horror – he's come over to say hello. *Except it never happens like that, does it?* No! So it's a good thing the Flirt Diva has come up with the nitty-gritty of Making an Approach.

Are you up for it? Ready to lay some Venus flirt-traps and broadcast that you are ready, willing and available? After all your efforts, you should be! But first let me ask you this. Have you ever made an approach on a guy? If so, bravo! If the answer however is no, I'd like to ask why not? Surely you cannot still be schlepping around waiting for a guy to saunter over or make a move on you? C'mon, that is *so* last century! If there's one thing I have learnt by now, it's that we have to smash the old rules in order to shimmy forward with the new.

Why is it so damn hard for us to make the first move? Am I being naive in clinging to the belief that 21$^{st}$ Century women are about sass, independence, equality and the ability to express themselves? Added to that, our vastly improved social and economic status means that professionally and financially, we're a gazillion times better off than our parents. *Wake up ladies.* We're living the dream! The downside is that, romantically, things are a little trickier. And by not executing a thoughtful *love* strategy, we are assuming that being a woman still means: *Waiting for a man to approach. Make the first move. Do all the work.* But ladies, that is not what the Flirt Diva is about. There's nothing sassy about being passive! Surely that kind of thinking is trapped back in the prehistoric era. Before we'd fought tooth and nail for a quality of life where equality is the norm? You can bang on all you like about the old hunter/gatherer/caveman thing, but excuse me, have we forgotten about Girl Power? Hmmm? So, no, things are not as simple as the olden days, it *is* more complicated today. Obviously in our parents' generation, women would never just rock up to a guy and holler "Oi big boy". But today, we get to write our own script and make our own rules. How lucky are we?

So before you come up with all the reasons you can't march up to a man with a sexy, confident approach, look him in the eye, dish out your most winning smile and introduce yourself – understand this – there is absolutely no shame in making an approach. Why the heck shouldn't we? What rule book says we can't? It's not 19-freaking-52! And anyway, making the first move is about pursuing someone because you really want them, not just because they happened to approach you.

So for the moment at least, it's time to revolutionise your Flirt Diva stance and become Ms Take-Charge – if you want to widen your love options that is. Just remember assertive – not aggressive. You're just pointing, clicking, smiling and saying "hi!" By doing that, you're giving him the green light to take things from there. And if we didn't do that, half the time nobody would be talking to anybody! Especially in the troubled political world in which we live, where we stride down the streets of the big cities and do our best to avoid eye contact. That won't cut it for the Flirt Diva, you need to PAY ATTENTION. Keep your radar finally tuned for guys who are friendly and above all non-threatening. They're just too easy to miss if you're not *focusing.*

And yes, I am aware it can be a nail-biting, stress inducing nightmare at first. Moreover there are no rejection-free routes, but remember that *both* your egos are central to the art of flirting. It's not just *your* ego at stake here, but your flirt-mates as well. Secondly this whole missive is about undertaking new challenges, correct? To get out there and road test the equipment. By now you should have built enough sturdy foundations that any rejections simply bounce right off you. Without a doubt, the best way to overcome the flirting heebie-jeebies is to go for *low risk situations.* You have absolutely nothing to lose *especially if you're never likely to see the guy again.* Word of warning though. The guy I'm talking about approaching is *not* Mr El Smootho and he's *not* a Player (we leave the Players well alone; they don't need us to help them along thanks).

The guy we're talking about is just your average cheeky chappy. He's a good guy. He's not chasing you, or everyone else in a skirt for that matter! He might be shy, or at the very least unsure about his sex appeal. But one thing's for sure, he's not a sleaze, and he's not about to put himself out there for rejection. "Fine!" you say. "Why should I?" The answer is simple. You're a Flirt Diva in training. You're going for gold. It's not your style to second guess anyone or short change yourself. You're becoming liberated. So really – where's the harm of shimming over and giving someone the green light by saying "hi"?

### Performance Anxiety

As you prepare to enter the gates of urban flirtification, you will need to be switched "ON" at all times. All set to turn up the vamp volume at a microsecond's notice and express yourself evocatively, exotically and hey, if it takes your fancy, *erotically.* Think of this as your first night opening at Vegas. Excuse me…you're nervous? Why? *Who's judging you?* This is no time to lose your nerves! Life's moving too fast. Just remember that confidence is key when it comes to unleashing your inner vamp and yours has been growing steadily. Agreed?

Likewise, when you pick up those droopy shoulders and swirl the ice in your drink oh-so seductively, you'll soon know what works and what doesn't. It's instinct.

You can do this. You know you can. You don't want to let yourself or your potential flirt-mates down. Nor do you want to risk being gossiped about in exclusive flirting members' circles because – you were too chicken shit to try. *Hell no!*

The adrenaline flows when we're keen to impress, in fact adrenaline in small quantities is mandatory for a sexually charged interaction. *"Yes"* I can hear you sniff. *"I learnt that when I was 12!"* Okay, fine smarty-pants, but when the simple act of just standing next to someone you're smitten with is enough to make you feel all moist and moochy – and temporarily screw with your speech patterns – it's happening for a reason. That reason is called 'lustiety'– lust and anxiety rolled into one. And you need to work with it, not against it!

No matter how confident you think you are, none of us are completely shock resistant. We can't avoid those klutzy moments. The one-liners that are thrown out into the wind and never quite caught. Just ask confidence queen Carrie Bradshaw who turned into a stammering fool every time she unexpectedly ran into Mr Big.

Eventually you will stop doing that thing where you analyse everything to death and blow it all out of all proportion. Like those times when you daydream about a future with some guy you met fifteen seconds ago! Why do women do that? And then they fast forward to plans about The Future before they even know anything about the guy; beyond his ability to stare out moodily from behind piercing blue eyes! Any wonder they feel the pressure if they carry on like that. *Sheesh!* The trick is to downplay your expectations when it comes to a night out, and therefore reduce your chances of getting struck down by the Curse of the Wobblies.

If you're feeling like Anxious Annie, plagued with fear on the left of you and panic on the right of you, it will show! So be prepared, and that way, if you *do* get stage fright, it doesn't have to screw everything up. It can actually help, in the same way that having wonky nerves can work to boost your confidence. It's just a matter of being *in control*.

At the end of the day, you're working hard to swathe yourself in concealable emotional body armour, so what's the problem? Put the ball in your flirt-mate's court and let him feel it, squeeze it, jiggle and tease it. *Boom, boom, boom*! Before you part ways, give him your toothiest smile and let him know that spending time with him was fun and – you'd like more. Just give him a sign already!

### And cut!

Finally a word about those demons and skeletons that can screw us up. They are real, they do exist and you will encounter them. But, wake up call ladies, rejection is a very real part of our lives, no matter whether your name is Jen Anniston or Plain Jane. It's not the rejection that's so fearsome, it's the *thought* of the rejection. And you can take all the Anti-Rejection Pills you want, but honestly, you'd be better off anticipating the worst case scenario because Sod's Law, it will happen!

Be equipped for the emotions that will hit and roll off you like thunder when you're out on the field. Prepare for a majestic explosion of every comical symptom of neurosis: anxiety, self-consciousness, vulnerability, impulsiveness, hostility. And don't even think about the violent stomach flips that will kick in the minute you step out of your comfort zone; or worse, when you try to strike up some chit-chat with someone you like – even just a teeny bit.

Be aware of the distorted messages your brain will send, as it fires off split second messages to undermine your bravado. It's usually right when you're about to make a move on Boy Wonder that Self-Sabotage makes a guest appearance. Look, here he is now with his big line: "*Hey! You can't talk to him. You don't have the balls.*" You know those nasty little voices, bought to you by the gremlins whose missive it is to stop you in your tracks, and talk you out of doing almost anything.

We'll call it CFS – Chronic Freak-Out Syndrome. Sufferers are typically *not in the habit* of making an approach, which explains why all these wild emotions rush to the surface and mess with us. There's only one thing to do. Keep your cool, remember to *breathe* and take stock of the situation. We've all been there. We've all experienced this heart attack inducing shite. You just have to stay calm. Switch your internal panic alarm off. Order a stiff drink and go forth on your mission. After showing courage of this magnitude, you deserve it!

So what happens if you point and click and make an approach but you trip up midway through your first line? Or you experience that long, awkward pause where you're just dying of embarrassment? I'll tell you what happens. Get over it! Your awkwardness is no worse than anyone else's. We all get the heebie-geebies – but what are you gonna' do? Just disregard it and crack on. That's what the pro's do. You don't see them take their bat and ball and go home when they fluff a line. Granted it's harder to twinkle 'n' flirt when your palms are sweaty, you just stood on his foot and your drink is sloshing all over the place. But hey, stay cool. Pretend it never happened.

"So" you ask "What do you do after you've given it your best shot but nothing's happening and if anything, it's all gone a bit weird?" The answer is simple – be honest with yourself. If you've been swerving daringly between shimmying shoulders and hair-flicking hip-rolling-moves, your hand brushing his seductively as you engage in some seriously sexy eye-contact – but getting no response then, ladies, hold your hands up in a surrender pose, deny and confirm nothing – and step away from the man! At this point it's fair to assume – he's just not that into you. Sorry for being harsh – I just don't want to see you wasting your time, and flirt juice.

*So long as you followed these 3 rules <u>before</u> you gave up the game:*

1. You waited for the right moment to corner him, not when he was in the middle of something else.
2. You were crystal clear with the signals you were sending out and repeated them frequently.
3. You were supremely confident that you delivered your signals with clarity and purpose – not in a `blink and you'll miss it' way.

If you did follow the flirt rules (and used practice and repetition to get your message across), and you gave it a good few minutes for the vibe to kick in, and he still didn't get it, then you have two choices. You can either invest your energy in someone more receptive (let's see if that doesn't get Mr I-Don't-Get-It's attention). Or, and this one's just for hardcore extremists, take one final plunge and ask, *"So dude, are you straight or gay?"* Kidding!

Failing that, the first law of getting out of an uncomfortable situation is to simply head back to base. If you really want to, you can glide by a little later and see where the land lies, but only if your flirtitution tells you it's the right thing to do. Not because you've downed nine Crack Baby shots in the past three and half minutes to give yourself the courage.

The key is not to take it too seriously. It's just fun and games – until someone loses an ego that is. Boo-hoo! But hey, it takes a true Flirt Diva disciple to get that maracas shaking message over the line and into his mind, but if anyone can do it, you can. *Keep telling yourself. Believe in yourself!*

And once you get the hang of it, you'll soon become addicted to the healthiest high you've ever had. Just watch and see.

### *So You've Been Rejected?*

Don't get me wrong, I understand the pain of rejection. Oh yes. I've been there. But hey, I lived to tell the tale – as will you. So let's just say things haven't gone as you'd hoped, and basically he's delivered the holy grail of the world's most tactless knock-back – it happens to the best of us – but how are you meant to cope? The trick is *not to take it personally.* Who knows what shit is going down with him! Perhaps he's just come off the Prozac or been dumped by his girlfriend of eight years; or maybe he's constipated. Either way, it is absolutely no reflection on you so *don't panic.* Just remember – emotional detachment.

Wretch out your Flirt SOS emergency toolbox, pop a peppermint and with a flick of your glossy hair; teeter off to the loo, zap on some perfume, pouf up your powder, shine up your lips and Flirt Diva, get back out there! If you do see him again, give him a gigantic grin. Don't let him know he's upset you, he's not worth it!

Now is the time to take a big breath. What is the worst thing that can happen if you make a move on someone and they kick you to the kerb? Take a moment to think about it. At the end of this section I'll ask you to write down the things that scare you the most when it comes to making an approach. As well as what you can do to help get over your fear of rejection, and get on with the task of being the superhero you know you can be. What is the basis of your fear? Losing face? Being turned down? Being fobbed off? I suspect it's a little of all of the above. We're only human. We all have feelings. We might like to be automated robots when it comes to this stuff, but we're not.

So what are you meant to do when the going gets tough? I'll tell you what you'll do. How about you roll with the punches and take it on the chin. We've got no real cause for fear. No-one can hurt us, well certainly no-one we have no emotional investment in. Save that energy. In the meanwhile, focus on making a meaningful bond with someone real, someone who appreciates you.

Anyway, who said all rejection was all bad? There will always be obstacles and challenges to overcome before the leading lady gets her man. Hello Mills & Boon! Or any romance novel, where emotional conflict meets inner turmoil. You know the drill. Girl meets boy. Boy backs off. Girl chases boy. Boy is a fuck-up and causes girl nothing but grief. Girl backs off. Boy cleans up his act. Girl takes him back. And there's your happy ending. It is genuinely baffling half the time, but somehow, the less sense it makes, the better it seems to work out in the end! So take the rejection on the chin because – who knows where it might lead.

So yes, you will experience bouts of Occasional Discomfort, Random Humiliation and Unexplained Rejection; and you will have to fight off that sickening feeling that comes with stage fright – but tough! Because do you know what? This is what makes the truly great Flirts. The rest are left on the sidelines. You're only as good as your last flirt-battle. If you went down in the line of fire, you need to pick yourself up, dust yourself down and Get Back Out There. Look at it this way; if you were brave enough to go to battle in the first place, you're brave enough to tackle that final frontier and Give Him a Sign. You can run but you can't hide. And so long as you've taken your shock resistant treatment and got your Flirt-Squad cheering you on for moral support, you'll be fine.

So if you've got your chat-pump ready, aimed and firing, but your flirt-mate isn't keeping up with you, and the conversation lacks any natural rhythm don't, I repeat, don't freak out. Help is at hand (if you've been an eager diva and done your homework that is!) Deal out your FFA – Fun, Friendly and Approachable cards, and play them at every opportunity. It's the natural way to help bring out the best in anyone. Then just reach into your vault and bring out some ice-breaker bits and bobs.

In fact the only mistake you can make, if you are feeling jittery or uncomfortable, is to hold back and bite your tongue for fear of making a twat of yourself. Who cares if you say the wrong thing, or snort rather too loudly when you laugh? No-one's testing you. No-one's grading you. This is not a life or death situation. You can bet your bottom pound your flirt-mate isn't perfect. *He's just some guy*, and if he's a wanker, you walk. So don't be shaking in your boots, obsessing about "how hot he is". That'll only turn you into Nervous Nelly and as a fellow Flirt Diva, we can't be having that.

So stop bitchin' and start bewitching, you're not out fighting a war, you're just looking for a half decent freakin' bloke who'll make your heart soar. And contrary to popular belief, my experience is that blokes are *trying*. I can practically hear your sharp intake of disbelief as I say that (and sure, it's pretty bleeding obvious that some *are trying* more than others) but it's worth giving them the benefit of the doubt. And if it turns out that they're not trying at all, then ladies, you know the drill. Step away from the man!

*Golden Rule:* Don't take it too seriously. Or as Samantha says with one arched eyebrow on *Sex and the City: "Slap on the armour and go through life enjoying men, but not expecting them to fill you up."*

### Don't resort to liquid courage

As tempting as it is to slam dunk three tequila shots before you go up to that hottie at the bar, you will ultimately find being sober-ish (or just slightly buzzed) is far more appealing (and productive) than being completely stonkered. It can be a bugger trying to keep that banter burning brightly when you're half sozzled – and yes, I would know! You'll be laughing too loudly and for too long because, ah, you've got no idea what to say next! And when your intoxicated brain settles on something totally outlandish to say – you'll come off even worse.

So let me put on my nanny hat, and ask you not to sell yourself short. Don't let your wit and charm get buried under too much booze. You'll be left stumbling and slurring your words, struggling to make a face that says, "I'm shnotas tipsee asyouthinkIam." Instead, practice summonsing up your courage while you've still got control of your faculties. A shot of Dutch courage never hurt anyone, but forget about necking too much of the hard stuff. You could come off much worse in the long term when you find you've got no control whatsoever. This of course, is when things start to go pear shaped.

*"Women over (in the U.S) there are very predatory, they're like, "When are you taking me out?" It's scary sometimes. I wasn't brought up to go up to guys and say, "So when are we having sex then?" I don't say anything, and in the meantime someone else has gone over there and I'm like, "Sh*t, what the f*ck? Give me two seconds here!"*

\- Estelle on living and loving in America

### Chapter 10. There's a male revolution going on... You read it here first

*"Is it true all men are freaks?"* asks Carrie in an early episode of *Sex and the City.* Happily, the Flirt Diva thinks not. They're not all freaks, but they are a little er, different to us and we're going to try to get our head around what's going on in theirs. So grab a cup of something hot, and settle in for hanky-panky happy hour.

For centuries, men have been begging us to just *tell them how we feel already!* Through a tradition of songs, poems and lyrics for centuries, so go on, throw him a bone. You don't have to come on all hot and heavy. Just give him a sign. There have been too many signal breakdowns between men and women over the past few decades and far too much good relationship potential screwed because of them.

And let's be honest, guys have Signal Failure all the time. They find it extremely difficult to tell the difference between a gal-pal who is simply being cute and friendly, and the babe who is trying to make a move on them. I'll bet my diamond encrusted eyelash that there's not a single one of you reading who hasn't been in the position of trying to let a friend know that you were interested in ah – more – but typically, he just did not pick up on that ole love vibe. So you went and lost your nerve, and as a result – you will never know whether he shared those feelings or not! How frustrating! The point is – guys *miss flirting signals* all the time! What you might think is really damn obvious is most probably not! In fact it most certainly isn't. You're thinking "He must know I want to shag him." He's thinking "It's cool how she's so friendly."

And it's not that surprising. You know how OCD men are with their maps and the need for sign-posting. They can't bear to ask for directions or instructions for fear of diminishing their manly pride. He doesn't have the best navigation tools when it comes to love though does he? No maps, charts or compass – nothing to give him any clue of what's on your mind. It's up to you to *give him directions.* You need to S.P.E.L.L I.T O.U.T.

Men aren't mind readers (much to our chagrin) and no matter how razor sharp you think his radar is, even when you're sending what you consider your hardest hitting signals, *don't expect him to get it.* And look, this is really tricky territory. It is a fine line between letting someone know you're hot for them and coming across like a total desperado, but generally speaking, women do tend to lean towards the subtle approach. And while I vehemently discourage anyone from unleashing slut tactics like er, grinding your leg into his crotch, you simply can't be too subtle either. Your efforts *will be lost.* You do need to bang that gorilla over the head to make your signals loud enough to be heard; otherwise they will go straight over his head!

*Uh-oh: Signal Breakdown folks. All passengers please disembark.*


### More man stuff

Let's talk about men's insecurities. Are they all screwed up when it comes to matters of the heart? Just as dazed and confused about the rules as we are? Too terrified to make an approach, because frankly, they've been burnt before?

In order to answer these questions and more, we really need to lift the lid on men's psyche to reveal the goings-on of their often bewildering behaviour. We all share the same insecurities when it comes to the big two – Sex and Rejection. So perhaps the first thing to say is that *of course* men share the same frustrations and fears as we do. They have different ways of expressing them but that's largely due to conditioning.

Since we were little girls, many of us, have been lucky enough to enjoy the depth and emotional support that women genetically tend to give

217

each other, whilst men have not. Traditionally we've had years of girly get-togethers and bonding sessions spent pouring over the luv-stuff. This was comfort food for the soul. It helped us cope with the crazy shit that we would invariably go through in adolescence and adulthood. We spent so much time mooching over boy stuff, pouring over the details in those endless angst-inducing sessions with our girlfriends. But it's a rare and lucky guy that has that level of connection with his mates. Which is why men are struggling to keep up, bless 'em.

The sad reality is that most guys don't have a clue about flirting. I know, I know, it's like, get with the program! Research carried out extensively in this field confirms that an alarming 3 out of 4 men have *no idea* that you are flirting with them. Is now the time to think about becoming bi-sexual? Maybe!

Let's look at the reasons behind it. Men don't have access to as much readily available information to help navigate them through these screwy times. Of course you could argue that the information is all there, they just have to go and find it, but in their defence, a greater portion of men are getting used to the idea of emotional support via self-development. They've started bandying around words like "bonding" and "quality time" and other such modern age-isms, which is great, but generally guys just don't have the benefit of our emotional wisdom – simply because they haven't been as resourceful in this area. But wait, there is some good news, if you surf the net or look through any lads' mags, you will find the same broad range of flirting tips as the ones you're reading here – and written by women. Hoorah!

So there's evidence that men *are* educating themselves about this stuff these days, even if it is only via the lads mags. But hey, it's better than nothing! Obviously it works to all of our advantages if blokes are armed

218

with the Flirting Translation handbook. And while they're not yet experts in the field, they are at the very least getting familiar with the signals they should be *looking out for*. This alone makes it easier for them to decode *our flirting system*. And thus makes your investment into Flirt Divadom all the more worthwhile!

Another fact I picked up from a scientific survey conducted at erm, my local boozer, is that guys *are* generally happy to admit that women are the superior sex when it comes to flirting prowess, which of course they love for the simple reason that it makes their job *less complicated*. The general consensus is that men prefer it when we make it nice and straightforward for them – no big surprise there.

Further scientific studies (which I've worked at tirelessly) reveal that the highest proportion of men go for take-charge women. They think confidence is dead sexy. Studies back it up with proof that men love being approached by women. This is where binge-flirting comes into play. It's about bombarding him, not in an OTT way, but with enough self-assurance that he simply cannot miss the message.

I'm not saying that men can't flirt, but ladies, I've studied the tools and rules and believe me, we're living in a world where women follow the rules and men *are* largely the tools!

Keep in mind there is a big difference between flirting with confidence, clarity, and sassiness as opposed to flirting in a silly, giggly or overtly sexual way. You do need to be aware of what you're doing so you don't come across as a man-eater, or just plain balmy. Remember, assertive not aggressive. Cooing over him like a sex object is one thing. Throwing him against the wall and sticking your tongue down his throat is quite another.

So when you find yourself in that familiar gut-churning situation, where it's just you and him, and you've got one chance – go for it! You are absolutely in the driving seat, so don't hold back. Flutter those lashes! Flick that hair! Fondle his arm! You'll know within the first ten minutes if he's hot for you or not.

And while I hate to make things sound more complicated than they really are, do be aware that while he might be going out of his way to be charming and friendly, he may *not* have any desire to drag you back to his cave. It could just mean he's flirting for fun, not for intent, which is exactly what we're learning to do here. So don't give him a hard time over it. Just try to gage whether this is his "friendly" persona, or if it somehow feels different. Listen to your gut. Always. It will rarely let you down – even when your bullshit detector stops working. At the end of the day it's our instinct we have to rely on. And if you find yourself thinking you'd have more chance of knowing where you stood with a dancing bear, then I can appreciate you asking, "What's a girl to do?"

### El-Smootho Vs The Shy Guy

Well, first up you need to know how to spot the difference. Because there are two kinds of guys you will encounter. There is the confident dude who is all clued up about this flirting lark, and there is the guy who's not. The Sammy Suave type will automatically think every woman is waiting to hit on him. He'll come across as attentive and assertive, his actions will be sharp and super focused. He'll be grinning like an alligator, ready to indulge in some "touchy-feely" and primed, like a beady-eyed hawk watching for your signals.

The shy guy on the other hand, will have a cute crooked smile glued to his face with glazed eyes, thinking, "Shit, I really like her", but be

220

pathologically clueless when it comes to what to do next. But you don't know that! Nor do you know if he's licking his wounds from the last violent apprehension he got when he so much as smiled at someone! So give him a break already!

And seriously, spare a thought for the bloke's point of view. They don't always get it easy. They've clocked up miles of experience when it comes to sexual rejection; they've been trod on and spat out. I'll be honest with you, I think it sucks that so many good men are getting such a hard time of it today. It doesn't help when women are so goddamn haughty. Look at it this way, if he's a philanderer, a serial sex-fiend or a complete and utter nutter, then yes, he deserves to be gotten rid of. But, if his only crime is that he had the audacity to *speak to you,* and you come down on him like a ton of bricks, it doesn't fare well for anyone. That's because he won't be making any more attempts on anyone again – ever! Not so good for the sisterhood 'ey?

### Babes in Boyland

Always keep in mind that you're dealing with the UFME – Ultra Fragile Male Ego – and as incredulous as it sounds, his ego may even be more delicate than yours. *No, stop it!* But seriously, he is not going to respond to any monkey business unless it's one hundred percent in the bag. He has to be *absolutely confident* about making a move and only when he is, will he take a chance. His Great Big Sensitive Male Ego will not let him get it wrong. That means having the full assault of your flirting artillery poised to target the bull's-eye. We're talking balance, accuracy, timing and vision. And when he does get it, you'll know about it. I can just see him swinging from the vine now; howling the blood curdling cry of Tarzan style lust.

So the *real* thrill of mutual flirting – besides kicking out a few *Kill Bill* style moves of your own – is that it allows you to interpret the signals you're getting back. That means you're already streets ahead *if* you've done your homework, because *you* know what you're looking for. Everything should look clearer now that you've studied the big players, and got some fresh insight into your own romantic escapades. This all helps in your bid to recognise the green light when it comes to figuring out whether Tommy Terrific fancies you.

Here's what you should be looking for to get some insight into how he's feeling. And I'll give you a tip, it's pretty much the same stuff we use, so it shouldn't be too hard to spot!

***You'll know you're in with a chance with these non-verbal cues:***
- The beer belly goes in and the shoulders go back as he *struts* across the room.
- He angles his body so he's facing you full frontal.
- He grins like a Cheshire cat. Every chuckle tells you – it's working!
- He keeps glancing over your way – up to three times or more.
- He's up for a dance.
- His mate simply vanishes.
- He says his going to the toilet – and he comes back.
- He gets that soft gooey look in his eye when he talks to you.
- He initiates a full body bear-hug when he says goodbye.
- He gives you the *Blue Steel* power stare.
- He dips an imaginary cap.
- His eyes twinkle with a naughty glint.

*Listen out for these <u>verbal</u> cues:*

- He over uses your name – a big, fat giveaway!
- He tells you something fun that he's doing tomorrow night.
- He compliments you – on anything at all.
- He talks about the bands, movies or restaurants he'd like to see and try.
- He tells you that being single is great, but…
- He makes an effort to talk (not flirt) with your buddies.
- He offers to buy you a drink.
- He gives you his phone number. D'oh!

OK, so what about the blokes? What are they looking for on the flirting floor: besides a wink, a wave and a smile? I checked out www.askmen.com website to see what advice those guys were dishing out for their lovelorn readers. I'm happy to say it's not too different to what we're dishing out here. Hoorah!

*"She held my glance for two seconds longer than normal in a way that signals to a hunter 'I want something from you'."*

- Boris Becker, former world championship tennis player (after an impromptu indiscretion in a broom closet.)

Here's their advice when it comes to what he's looking for. *See how many you can tick off*:

1. You make the initial approach.
2. You invade his personal space.
3. You make extended eye-contact.
4. You play with your hair.
5. You play with his hair.
6. You mimic his body movements.
7. You isolate yourself from your friends.
8. You draw attention to your mouth, your neck, your breasts.
9. You walk by and look back over your shoulder.
10. You play the "touchy feelies" with his hand, his arm – his whatever!

And look, you might think some of these are a tad obvious, so here at Flirt Diva HQ, we've come up with one that he might find slightly more obscure:

You pull him in close, push him up against the wall and lunge in for that lip bruising tongue crushing kiss you've been longing for. *He'll never know what's on your mind!*

### What should *you* be looking for?

It's useful to know what signals and clues *the blokes* are dishing out. And since we've established that most of what we communicate is via our body language, we need to know what his body is *really* saying. The bonus is that while you're busy watching for clues, you'll become less self-conscious about your own performance – but still as focused of course!

***Right then, what should he be doing to show he's keen?***

*Are you kidding?*

- He should use the furry warmth of his hand to wipe the raindrop from your face.
- He should be sighing "I could get used to this" as he peels you a grape and brings you another glass of champagne.
- He should be using his eyes to devour your lips, your hips and laughing like a madman at your wit.
- He should hold your eye-contact intensely: heat-seeking eyes asking tough questions and looking for answers!

***Or, he could simply use any of these top giveaways:***

1. Eyebrow flash: He raises one or both eyebrows pantomime style for a couple of seconds, followed by a rapid lowering to the normal position. (Otherwise known as the brow-bobbing bloke). The flash is often combined with a smile and strong eye contact. This indicates a cheeky and often suggestive message!

2. Lip lick: Very common. We unconsciously draw attention to our mouth if we're physically attracted to someone – and we want to suck their face off! It might be a single lip-lick, wetting the upper or lower lip, or running the tongue around the entire lip area. Whichever it is, he's thinking about what he'd like to do with your lips.

3. Short darting glances: Usually occurring in sets, with an average of 3 glances each for 3-5 seconds long. He lets you catch him looking and then he does it again. Cheeky bugger!

4. Hair flip: Or the male equivalent, he pushes his fingers through his hair, strokes his beard or plays with his 'tache. Either way he's got the heebie-jeebies bad and just *cannot* keep his hands still!

5. Half smile: He gives you a sort of half-smile, combined with serious eye contact so direct it drills right into your soul. *He is telling you he's in lust with you!*

6. Whisper: He leans over and speaks oh so softly into your ear and creates a secret intimate world just for the two of you. *Mmmmm.*

7. Primping, preening or peacocking: He pats or smoothes down his clothing even if it doesn't need any adjusting. *He wants to look his best for you.*

8. Shirt sleeve hike: The top of the shirt sleeve goes up to expose a little more of that forearm. *What a show off!*

9. He puts his hands on his hips or in his belt loops to accentuate his nether regions. *Showing you the goods!*

10. Object caress: He manhandles his keys, drums his fingers up and down, plays with his lighter or anything he can find to wrap his mitts around - *in lieu of you.*

11. Leg opener: He opens those legs even wider. *Phwoar.*

12. Posture: The way he's sitting and standing becomes more er, erect. *Say no more.*

13. Secret gaze: He looks at you like he's seeing you for the first time. *He thinks he could love you*

14. Undivided Attention: He ignores the Pammy Anderson style blonde over in the corner. *Because no-one compares to you!*

### *Right back at ya*

OK, so what about you? What are you saying and is *your message clear*? Or has it become muddled through the puddle of sexual politics? Don't let it. Let your body do the talking! Sexual attraction is all about communicating and receiving signals with hot body language and killer eye-contact. Whether it's the way you lower your voice, the curve of your smile, or the tilt of your adorable head – you're transmitting a very sexy message. Get more power behind your message by using everything you've got!

**What he's looking for from you:**

- A big, open mouthed toothy smile.
- A fun game of "touchy feelies".
- Eyebrows raised and then lowered, followed by a sexy smile.
- Straight, upright posture where everything appears firmer and tauter.
- Laughter in unison and then – drum roll – an exchange of eye contact in acknowledgment of 'the moment'.
- Rubbing your wrists up and down with your thumb and forefinger very slowly.
- Gazing into his eyes with a lazy, half smile.
- Rocking back and forth towards him – targeting him fair and square.
- Raising or lowering the volume of your voice to match his.
- Rubbing your chin or touching your cheek or lips – indicating you might like to touch him this way!
- Biting your lips, showing your tongue, licking your lips.
- Twirling your hair around your fingers while exchanging smouldering eye-contact.
- Giving compliments. Loads of them!

**How do I get the Mills & Boon: I'm making `eyes' at you...?**

Without a doubt *the most potent flirting tool we have is our eyes.* Eye-contact is the most direct way to signal to what's really on your mind. It's a simple gesture that can open up the floodgates for some real, raw emotion.

The power of the penetrating gaze should never be underestimated. There's a reason they call our eyes the windows to our soul – even blokes get it!

A lingering look from a foxy lady like yourself, is literally a green light. It's even more effective if you "think" the thought while you transmit the look. For example, if you want to send a sensual message, simply think sexy thoughts while you're making eye-contact. Hold his eye contact for a split-second too long before slowly, unwillingly pulling away. Repeat after fifteen seconds. Let your eyes reveal everything – or nothing. Just be aware of their power and start using them to their full potential. You'll get a chance to practice in Day 2 of the challenges.

***Blow Him Out of His Sox*** *Flirting Tip #1 The cheeky smile*
The ladies known as the super Angels: Drew Barrymore, Cameron Diaz and Lucy Liu are famous for their miles of cheeky smiles. Care to give it a try next time Boy Wonder saunters over and says, *"Alright Gels?"*
But remember it only works if you do these two things:
1) Make sure your smile reaches all the way to your eyes – work those crows' feet!
2) Use your eyes to communicate your sultry, "sex face." C'mon, you know how to do it!
***Top Tip:*** *Smile in a mysterious and secretive way, and make it clear that you are aware of, and very much in favour of, the sexual tension going on here.*
*What's the best way to do that?*
Get your Flirt Squad to cheer and whoop in the background
*Kidding!*

Much better to…


**Blow Him Out of His Sox** *Flirting Tip #2*

Practice the peek-a-boo. You can do it face-to-face or from a distance. Everyone loves the tantalizing feeling of being "peeped-at".

*Top Tip*: Keep your lips pursed and your head still. Tilt your head ever so slightly when you smile. Lower your eyes and hit him with the full force of your oh-so seductive gaze.

Give it a try now. Go on!


**Blow Him Out of His Sox** *Flirting Tip #3*

The raised brow with a slash of oo-er naughtiness thrown in.

This time we'll call on Ms Jolie – high priestess of the brow flash.

*Top Tip: Use this in conjunction with the cheeky smile as described above. Just every now and again though, you don't want to look like a drunk and disorderly clown.*


***Turn up the vamp volume and sex up your sound-nique***

*Think of your voice as a seduction tool. That's not you talking manically with the gasps and screeches is it? No! You've been practicing your sexy voice and now it sounds like dripping honey – all amber hues and sultry blues.*

- Learn to give great voice, think *sounds of seduction!*
- Listen to Hollywood's greatest. Marilyn, Garbo, Harlow, Bacall.
- Use a low, soothing voice and monitor your inflexions (you don't want to be sending anyone to sleep with your dull monotone).
- Lower your voice and create a "secret circle" where only *he* can hear.

- Lean in and whisper, brush his arm then pull away – ooh-er you little wildcat!
- Let out a long deep sigh.
- Make purring sounds.
- Communicate with energy!

### Whispering Sweet Muffins

Reach for your inner babeness – no shouting please! Take in his neck, his jaw, his Worzel Gummidge hairline! Let your sweet minty breath blow softly in his ear as you titter in-between sentences. Think you can do that? He'll think you're some kind of goddess if you can.

### Arm and hand-nique. Think Belly dancing.  Think sex. Think Shakira!

Graceful hand movements can be mesmerizing, not to mention highly *erotic*. Well, we all know what a good set of hands can do for a man…Hmmm? Flaunt yours lavishly when you're in full storytelling mode. Let your beautifully manicured nails shimmer and sparkle while your dancing fingers illustrate a story as melodiously as if you were playing the piano. Drum your fingers on the table to bring attention to sculpted hands and delicate wrists.

### Head & Shoulders

- Wear a low hanging necklace that settles tantalisingly in your décolleté.
- Find your best profile and use it.
- Cup your chin in your hands in a classic Audrey Hepburn pose

***Leg-nique: Think Naomi Campbell (when she's not spitting in policemen's faces)***

- Rest your hands under your legs.
- Slide your foot in and out of a backless shoe.

## *Nice and Easy*

Touching and rearranging someone can be lovely, provided you do it with *finesse*. In other words, don't just grab him! Gently warn him that you're moving in nice and slowly. Say it's his tie that you're aiming for, first pat the area gently with your hand *before* you do the adjusting. There's nothing worse than being grabbed by someone when you're not expecting it; much better to think like a predator. A proper jungle tigress will find her target, gather up all her powers of concentration and then silently move in for the kill. *Grrrr!*

## *Flirt Baby Flirt*

Of course there will be days you don't feel like flirting, but do it anyway and just see how you go. You might be surprised how much better you feel once it clicks in. If it doesn't, go home and read a good book. You don't have to beat yourself up about it. Best selling author and sexpert, Tracy Cox recommends in her book *Hot Sex* that you have sex (with your partner) even if you don't feel like it! Her theory is to give it a go and see how you feel once you get started. Well if it's good enough for sex – it's good enough for flirting!

***5 instant Fix Its, guaranteed to sort out any teething problems:***

- Breathe
- Stand tall
- Make eye-contact
- Be approachable
- Smile!

### Do the bootyshake

And listen up, once you hit the dance-floor to shake those hips and be all sexy-like, don't forget to *smile*. Otherwise what could happen is that you're looking so damn sexy and hot with those moves and that pout – that he gets all intimated by your unassailable beauty and runs away – it happens! Be sexy by all means, but keep it light and fun – in other words – non-threatening!

### As the evening comes to a close

You really need to pay close attention. Watch the signals, the body language and most especially his *eyes*, to see whether you qualify for his, "I'm Hot for You!" short-list. It's all part of the Get Loved Up flirting machine. Come on, you should know this stuff off by now!

### Oh, sod off!

We've all been the subject of unwanted attention by unwelcome cretins who will try it on with anyone. At some point you will encounter the lowlifes' out there. That arrogant, obnoxious dude who we've all had the dreariness of dealing with (their definition of flirting is somewhat questionable – hissing sounds anyone?). So if he's morphed from a sweetie into psycho, or he's leaping all over you like a lecherous glob, pitching out lines like: *"I think you should know my specialty is sexual harassment."* There are a couple of exit hatches:

- You can fake an emergency phone call. Simply excuse yourself as you swing your phone up to your ear and concentrate hard - just hope it doesn't ring!

- Fall back on the exit speech you prepared earlier and get set to make your speedy Gonzalez escape. The practised Flirt Diva has an escape hatch ready at all times to deal with unwanted attention, but, blessed is she who remembers her manners. Provided the guy's not wearing a *Slipknot* mask and singing, *my ding-a-ling, my ding-a-ling, won't you play with my ding-a-ling* it doesn't hurt to be graceful in your rejection.

**What you should not say is:**

*"Look Barry, Garry, Larry whatever your name is, I'm not interested, fuck off!"*

Or,

*"You wish jellyfish! Not a chance in Hell. On your scooter pooper!"*

What you *should* say in a friendly but firm tone is:

*"So, did you come here straight from Idiot Island tonight?"*

Just kidding!

What you should **really** say is:

*"Don't be such a whiny little bitch!"*

Kidding!

*Seriously, what you should say is:*

*"Look Barry, thanks for the compliment but I have to go. Goodbye!"*

## Drawing up the Flirt Zones

You can flirt anywhere, so it makes sense to test *all the flirting hotspots*. In terms of the most obvious places, flirt-ortunities are of course rampant in bars, clubs and well, anywhere there's entertainment and alcohol really (it's amazing what alcohol can do to loosen up the flirting muscle). So while it may be wholly unoriginal, it does make sense to start your flirting foray in a bar type environment. That way you get a chance to ogle others as they flirt: observe and learn – and then dazzle all and sundry with your fancy-pants new skills.

But why not try to be abstract in your bid to reach bloke heaven. Certainly according to the world of *Sex and the City,* it can happen anywhere. You can meet a honey while you're out buying food, riding the tube, playing darts or tossing a ball in the park. You can meet him while he's in his car, or at the bar, walking his dog or chopping a log. Get the idea? It's entirely up to you and your imagination.

Make it your mission to take in frenzied flirt-fests everywhere. But rather than going out with the sole intention to "pull" which puts way too much pressure on the situation, concentrate instead on finding a setting where there is plenty of other activities or cool stuff going on – pool, pinball or live music performances. You're more likely to hook up with new people if you're chatting around the pool table, jumping in for a game of table-football, or MC'ing the juke box. That's what men do. You don't see them sitting through six hour bitchathons. They make plans to do stuff. So should you.

As a fully focused man seeking missile, you're likely to go through that stage where your entire focus is directed at places that are full of potential totty. But don't be knocking back invitations from pals for a trip to the museum, the movies or the theatre (on the basis you'll never meet anyone while you're fumbling through the dark and dusty auditoriums). And opt instead to knock back vats of vino in some dive called *Bar Idiot* with your mate, who will not stop bitching about her boss. It's boring, it's repetitive and it doesn't do either of you any good. This is why you must stray outside the no-brainer flirt-zones, like bars and clubs, it's the only way you'll broaden your horizons. Don't let your heart and hormones dictate where you spend your free time. Go anywhere and everywhere – regardless of its potential. You already know that Boy Wonder *always* turns up where and when you least expect him, so why get all tied up in knots bending over backwards to find him? When all you have to do is widen your horizons – and he will come.

### Playing the dating game

Since we've established that it's no longer relevant to depend on the old fashioned "chance" meeting with our soul mate, it does makes sense to exploit the techno-obsessed-world in which we live. A place where PC's masquerade as love machines, and open up the erotically explosive world of online dating.

Cyber dating (and flirting) has pretty much become a way of life for many. It's hard to resist when there's so much choice. It is a massive industry and sometimes overwhelmingly tacky. But the sheer convenience of rocking back in the comfort of our homes and evoking a gargantuan sexual smorgasbord with a clickedy click, click of our fingers can be hard to resist. Especially since we've found ourselves in a technosexual generation where a large portion of single (and not so single) folk have become steadfastly hooked on virtual dating and no-strings rendezvous. A massive machine spanning friends with benefits, fuck buddies and oodles of casual

235

sex!

At the end of the day, there is plenty going on in singles' land, certainly enough that you can mix it all up and, if you're armed with the right attitude, get out there and have a ball. Whether that's with speed dating, wine tastings, book readings, parties, events or holidays. If you're one of those girls' who's always turned your nose up at these dating options – maybe you could reconsider and give it a chance? If only for novelty value. It could be the difference between sitting at home scoffing chocolates, or out having fun with likeminded people – and if it doesn't work out, no-one says you have to stick around, but I bet you'll get some good dinner party fodder out of the experience!

The trick is to think of these opportunities as practice grounds, not *hunting grounds*. Your intentions are not specifically to meet the man of your life. You're out there to have fun and to roadtest your new found skills on real life people – and just maybe, a red hot man!

Having said that, it's good to keep things in perspective, there is some pretty wacky stuff going on out there. There are websites for every taste, from super straight to really freaky; many of which are no doubt frankly dodgy. But if you do fancy getting involved with the sometimes ominous, but always entertaining, world of online dating, there will be a website that suits your criteria perfectly. Having said that, I'm not sure how confident I'd feel about weighting up my love life based solely on a psychic reading or "love" guidance dished up by a spiritualist's intuition, but by all means go ahead and try it, if that's what floats your boat.

Generally speaking when it comes to dating choices and experimentation, you'd be best to lose your prejudices. And while you're there, lose the sour faced friends as well. The ones who will shoot you down in flames the minute you say you're going to try something new. It's alright for them to pooh-pooh it, they're probably all loved up in their nice cosy relationships. Oh sure, they'll tell you online dating is crap, or it's "not your style" but you're not doing it for them. You're doing it to cast your net wider. It just makes practical sense. You're multiplying your chances of meeting new people, and frankly where else are you supposed to meet them? At work? I don't think so. At your regular haunts? Unlikely. Through friends of friends? Erm, maybe. So don't be listening to anyone's negativity. Tell them it's a shame they don't approve, but you're doing whatever it takes to have a happy fulfilling life, so why don't they respect that, and encourage you. Or sod off.

### *Stepping out onto the field*

Right then, in order to exercise your freshly developed flirt muscle and sharpen the tools of your trade, you will now study and *memorize* each of the following Pick 'n Mix Binge-Flirt moves and grooves, in a bid to lock them down. The challenge is to have them ready to access 24/7, as and when the flirt-ortunities arise. And they will, my Flirt Diva, they will.

♥       ♥       ♥

**Day 1.** The Pick 'n' Mix Binge-Flirt.

**Day 2.** Eye contact.

**Day 3**. Integrating with your day-to-day.

**Day 4**. Reading the signals.

**Day 5.** Dealing with rejection.

**Day 6.** Dating games.

**Day 7.** Spot-check!

## DAY 1

## THE PICK ''N' MIX BINGE-FLIRT

Right then, drum-roll please, I'd like to introduce the 3 x 3 Pick 'n' Mix, otherwise known as the Binge-Flirt *Boom, Boom, Boom!* This is where you select your favourite flirt gestures and assign your signature style. Once you've done that, prepare to bedazzle! You will do this simply by using your preferred gestures several times over, during the course of one or more electrifying flirt sessions. A three-minute exchange is all you need to get the party started. Scientifically, it's foolproof. Romantically, it's hot!

It's time to put your flirt mojo into overdrive. There's no room for one-trick ponies here. Boys will swoon, girls will flee, and you Ms Flirt Diva, will begin kicking serious butt on the flirt floor!

The first thing to do is to go through the *Pick 'n' Mix* selection below and find your signature style. Remember the key words – practice and repetition. Run through the moves until you've got your selection of a minimum of three down pat, and try out as many as you can in real life. Some of them you may find blindingly obvious, but don't let that put you off – that's the beauty of it – it is straightforward! Think monkey-see, monkey-do and mimic your flirt-mate's body language (subtly of course) and then just be fluid, natural and sexy – you know the drill!

Use every opportunity to bash out your moves, yes even during perfectly platonic conversations, (clearly this relates only to the "friendly gestures", not the overtly sexual ones. No teasing now!). Practice with colleagues, constables and cute boys. Pay attention to the impact you're having so you can be the judge of what works best. Get used to the art of being tactile. Nuzzle, touch, flick, sizzle and pop. This is no time to be shy or self-conscious, you're simply learning how to put on the razzle and dazzle. You'll have an absolute hoot when you're out doing this with your Flirt Squad.

The secret to developing your signature style is in knowing which gestures work specifically *for you*. It's no good wiggling your eye-brows in a seductive la Jolie fashion if you're a sweet, smiley girl at heart. It will just look silly. Likewise if you're the serious type, you can't lapse into a Girls Aloud giggle-thon – you've got to keep it real. Stay true to who you are, just amp it up a bit and keep your eye on the main prize – becoming a sexier, saucier, sassier version of yourself.

Once you've gone through the list and selected your armoury, it will be the most natural thing in the world to bring your gestures into play. You won't even have to think about it. You will always be on high flirt-alert and have your moves at top of mind, ready to pull out with effortless charm whenever you find yourself suddenly and unexpectedly – in the spotlight!

You will be kicking out impromptu flirting frenzies left right and centre. And the beauty of it is, you'll never be caught short again – we've all been there, haven't we? Sanding with your mouth gaping open wondering what the hell to do when you find yourself in the presence of the Omigod! guy. So, rather than clamming up, you'll be ready to take aim and fire! That's when you'll really start to appreciate your flirting prowess. Shining like the Queen of freakin' Sheba!

First up, think back to the Celebrity Flirt Styles we identified in Step 2. Just to recap they were:

- ❖ *Sweet Girly flirt*
- ❖ *Cheeky Flirt*
- ❖ *Mysterious flirt*
- ❖ *Hard and Fast flirt*
- ❖ *Tough Love flirt*

*OK, now take a look through the following list and tick <u>each</u> and <u>every</u> gesture that you just know you can pull off. Tick as many as you like, the more the merrier:*

*Arms:*

a. Hold your arms together as though you're lightly hugging yourself.

b. Put your arm around his neck and squeeze his shoulder.

c. Stretch sexily upwards, with your arms coming right back to rest behind your head.

d. Spread your arms open wide in a "come and get me big boy" kind of way!

e. Grab his hand in yours and say, "let's get out of here!"

*Eye-contact:*

a. Wink at him!

a. Lower your eyelids and flutter those lashes.

a. Give him the full beam of your glossy eyes and most attentive gaze.

b. Look him in square in the eye and deliver a sexy, breathy "thank you!" when he buys you a drink.

241

b. Give him a second – and a third – glance as he walks by.

b. Look him slowly up and down when he arrives to meet you and *then* give him your biggest smile.

c. Gaze at him thoughtfully, like you're trying to get inside his head.

c. Drop your gaze to his body and let your eyes take it all in slowly.

c. Peek at him over the rim of your glass.

c. Look at him for just a moment to long, then drop your eyelids and look mysteriously away in the distance.

d. Survey his face in close-up. Look at his stubble, the lines around his eyes, his forehead his mouth.

d. Drop your gaze to his lips and hold it there for five seconds. Then lift your eyes back to his.

d. Raise your brows suggestively as though to say, "hmmm, very impressive!" when he says something interesting.

e. Hold your eyebrows in the raised position until you get the response you want.

e. Think sexy thoughts and let those bedroom eyes turn to shimmering liquid before you tell him what you'd really like to "do tonight."

e. Gaze right into his eyes as you take his hand indicating it's, "time to go…"

### Head/Neck

a. Put your head on his shoulders in a mock demonstration of feeling sleepy.

a. Rest your cheek in your hands as you shower the full beam of your attention on him.

b. Cock your head towards his and lean in nice and close as you listen on high alert.

b. Look over your shoulder and give him a big juicy wink as you wander off.

c. Throw your head back and laugh rapturously at something he said

b. Tilt your ear towards his mouth and turn your face slowly towards his in a bid to "hear" what he's saying.

d. Expose the bare nape of your neck and massage it oh so slowly– very sexy.

e. Put your head between his legs and…Kidding! Move your face right in nice and close to his and ask him *anything* you want…


## Shoulders/décolleté

a. Sit upright and tilt your upper body towards him, facing him and leaning slightly forward.

b. Do a little shoulder shimmy in time to the music.

c. Combine a slow, lazy smile with a sexy shoulder shrug when he asks you a question that you'd rather not answer.

c. Tilt your head and tap your index finger on your ear to indicate that he speaks right into it.

d. Twirl that necklace, the one that's nestling snugly your décolleté.

d. Rearrange your neckline

e. Rest on both elbows on the table or bar, in a cocky "I own the joint fashion."

e. Pull up a reticent bra strap and give him a look that says, *"I'd be so much more comfortable without this on."*

### *Hips/legs/feet*: *Sitting*

a. Swing your legs from the bar stool.

a. Angle your foot towards his so they're almost touching, but not quite!

b. Play footsies and 'accidentally' graze his leg with your foot.

c. Sit with your legs underneath you and then, with all the allure you can master, uncoil them just at the right moment, extending them to their utmost length.

c. Cross your legs and draw little circles in the air with your foot (to highlight the calf muscle)

d. Twine your lower legs to flex your calf and flash that throbbing muscle.

e. Smooth your skirt seductively down over your thighs.

e. Do a *Basic Instinct* by crossing and uncrossing your legs, very slowly and very purposefully – if you dare!

### *Hips/legs/feet*: *Standing*

a. Shift your body weight from one foot to the other to result in subtly swinging hips.

b. Slap your thigh for dramatic effect when you laugh – even better his!

c. Roll those hips as you're walking away – just assume he's checking you out from behind.

d. Point your whole lower body towards his, with your upper body almost grazing his when you lean over to talk.

e. Stand facing him with your hands on your hips – if ever there was a time to say, *"how about it?"* this is it!

### *Hands/fingers*

a. Wave him over with an open handed circular gesture.

a. Give him a playful wave over your shoulder as you're walking away.

a. Sit with your hands demurely in your lap, but let your expression say something far cheekier

a. Fluff your hair and fiddle ever so slightly with your clothes.

a. Pat his shoulder when he says something clever, funny or just anything at all really.

a. Gesticulate (and use your perfectly manicured fingers to draw stories in the air).

b. Hold your hands up in the "I surrender" pose.

b. Tap him on the back or shoulder as he walks away and give him your most orgasmic smile.

b. Give him a "high-five!"

c. Use your index finger to touch-up your lip-gloss – right there in front of him.

c. Look left and right as though you're about to tell him a secret and use your index finger to beckon him closer.

c. Expose your palms and wrists (traditionally considered a highly erroneous zone).

e. Let your fingers trace the rim of your glass

c. Cup your hand over his as he lights your cigarette.

c. Make a steeple shape with your fingers and rest your chin on it

c. Hold your palms facing outward whilst telling him something personal

c. Use your fingers to draw a shape in the air and see if he can guess what it is

d. Tap your fingers against your upper thighs in time to the music.

d. Slide your palms slowly up and down across your lower thighs.

d. Clamp both hands on your thighs in a *"Good Lord if you only knew what I was thinking"* kind of way.

e. Put your hand out for assistance as you get up from your chair, then pull him in a little closer, if you've got anything intimate to say – now's the time!

e. Touch yourself, yes you heard me, stroke your throat, rub your neck, anything to show what a tactile creature you are.

e. Place your hands on both his shoulders and look him right in the face as you tell him what's on your mind.

## *Hair:*

a. Twirl your hair around your finger.

b. Flick that hair.

c. Shake your hair seductively out of its pony-tail and toss it all about.

d. Lift your hair up off your nape and pile it high on top of your head.

e. Tilt your head upside down and then flick it back in the manner of a rock star as you suggest something you could both do "later on".

## *Smile:*

a. Give him your sexiest shy-girl smile – all teeth and twinkly eyes.

b. Exercise every variation of the smile you can muster, from cheeky to seductive to snog-me-senseless.

c. Smile when you dance.

d. Hit him with your most seductive smile – make it long and slow and very deliberate.

e. Wait until the moment is just right to unveil your "secret" smile and then, tell him something that he's sure to remember.

*Mouth:*

a. Put your index finger in your mouth.

a. Make a small 'O' with your mouth in a "shocked" response to something he's said.

b. Pout teasingly.

b. Poke your tongue out (friendly not pornographic!)

b. Kiss his nose.

c. Blow him a kiss.

c. Keep your lips glossy, moist and kissable by licking them.

d. Mime something naughty and see if he can guess what it is.

d. Blow oh so softly into his ear.

d. Get in nice and close to his ear to tell him something and 'accidentally' nuzzle it.

e. Mouth the words to a terribly naughty song.

e. Take your straw out of the glass and delicately suck the end dry whilst looking right into his eyes.

*Full body:*

a. Whirl around on the pavement with your dress swirling about you ala Marilyn Monroe.

a. Put both your hands on his shoulders and sway your hips.

a. Shiver a little on a chilly night and move in nice and close.

b. Give him a sudden, quick blink-and-you-miss-it goodbye hug.

c. Brush lightly against his chest or torso and quickly move away.

d. Expose your arms, calves, belly or back.

d. Put your hand on your hip and press your elbow back for maximum chest pronunciation.

d. Accentuate your hotter than hot body part(s).

e. Stand with your feet apart, hand on your hips and lean in nice and close.

e. Say you're ready to call it a night and stand up and do a full body stretch. Now would be the perfect time to ask if he'll be "joining you."


***"Touchy Feelies":***

a. Straighten his tie, his collar or pick a bit of fluff from his jacket.

a. Cup his face in your hands and kiss both his cheeks.

b. Place your hand on his arm, his hand, his leg, his shoulder.

b. Play with his hair.

b. Play-punch his arm.

b. Tap his leg with your drink bottle.

b. Press his wrist in your hand to "check the time".

b. Hold his arm for just a moment and squeeze it while you make your point.

c. Wipe a fallen lash from his cheek.

d. Take his face in both your hands as you kiss his cheek goodbye.

e. Run both hands across his shoulders and forearms as you admire his shirt.

e. Put one hand on his waist as you kiss him goodnight.

e. Skim your hands lightly down his chest as you prepare to leave.

e. Pat him on the bum!


***Verbal:***

a. Invite him somewhere on impulse.

a. At the end of the night say: "I don't know this area; I'm totally in your hands".

b. Tell him, "I'll bet there's loads of girls' who fancy the pants off you".

b. Tell him he's got an "evil streak!"

b. Ask him if you can "read his palm" and take his hand in yours.

b. Tell him you haven't laughed so much in ages.

c. Say, "it's complicated" when he asks you for more information than you're prepared to give.

c. Tell him you've given up smoking and ask him to "blow smoke into your mouth".

c. Give him lots of long "Mmmmm" and "Mmm-hmm" sounds and low sighs when he's talking to you.

d. Tell him you think, "We should dance".

e. Turn to him after being interrupted and say: "I'm all yours now".

e. Ask him to hold still while you administer an intravenous love potion.


### Accessories:

a. Take out your compact mirror and fluff your hair.

a. Ask his taste in music, take out your iPod, cue up a song, pass him an earplug and exchange goo-goo eyes as you listen together.

a. Stir those ice-cubes lovingly around in your glass while giving him great eye-contact.

a. Raise your glass and make a toast to "the both of you." Chin, chin!

b. Play with his stuff: cufflinks, tie, water bottle, keys – anything that's not nailed down.

b. Offer him a sip of your drink.

b. Spray some perfume on your wrist and ask him to smell it.

b. Ask if he likes your necklace (and watch it create havoc as it points dangerously downwards!)

b. Use your feather hair accessory to tickle his nose.

b. Whip out your phone and take a candid photo of him.

c. Cool yourself down with an Oriental hand fan while you peek seductively over the top.

c. Strum your bangles and run them up and down your arm.

c. Dab a splotch of hand-cream onto his hand and rub it in oh so sensually while holding very steady eye-contact.

d. Readjust your shoulder bag across your chest.

d. Come back from the bar with 2 glasses of champers and make a toast to "tonight!"

d. Adjust your top.

d. Keep those phallic accessories close by and play with the stem of your wine glass, fondle that lighter and stroke that Bacardi Breezer bottle!

d. Lick that ice-cream.

d. Take off your scarf and pretend it's a whip.

d. Tap his leg playfully with your umbrella.

d. Give him 40 pence so he can "call you sometime!"

e. Ravish a banana – and ask if he'd like to know `how the banana felt'.

e. Juggle your little rubber ball (the must have flirting accessory – a girl's got to have balls).

e. Stand up and adjust your belt.

e. Offer to share your ice-cube with him and pop it half-way out of your mouth

e. Lean in to give him a kiss and squirt a mouthful of champagne into his mouth.

### If you picked mostly A's you're the Sweet Girly Flirt

*Signature flirt:* You are *the* princess. Prim and proper; a real prom queen. All big eyes and innocent smiles. You can be a little naïve when it comes to romantic stuff, but that just adds to your appeal. You play up your femininity – and guys absolutely love you for it!

*Flirting style:* Demure, ditzy, adorable, sweet, girly – with the ability to pull out some incredibly erotic shocks.

*Famous for*: Your sexual naivety, your love of romance and your quest for eternal love.

*Deadly weapon*: Glossy eyes, shiny smile and loads of cute outfits!

*If you were a drink, you'd be*: A big, creamy Kahlua and Milk.

*Movie star from another time:* Doris Day

*Just to recap your Sex and the City match is: Charlotte*

*Your A-List match is:* Cheryl Cole, Gwen Stefani, Kelly Brook, Duffy, Beyoncé, Jennifer Aniston, Terry Hatcher, Mischa Barton, Jennifer Hudson, Holly Willoughby.


### If you picked mostly B's you're the Cheeky Flirt

*Signature style:* You've got your own brand of cheeky brash innocence. You're quirky, sassy and forthright. You know how to win guys' over with that quizzical head tilt, the perfectly-timed hair flick, your incredibly sexy laugh, big-eyed gaze and attention grabbing wardrobe.

*Flirting style:* Touchy-feely with theatrical hand gestures and an irresistible OTT friendliness.

*Qualities:* Self-depreciating humour, you're not afraid to laugh at yourself and have a gag at your own expense. You're definitely the most fun flirt!

*Famous for:* You love to tease – in fact you can't help it – but it's usually harmless enough. You've got a cute and lovable personality combined with fearless fashion sense and you know how to push out the eyebrow-raising antics when you want to make an impact.

*Deadly weapon:* Big eyes. Soft fluffy hair. Disarming smile.

*If you were a drink, you'd be:* A glass of the finest champagne.

*Movie star from another time:* Audrey Hepburn.

*Just to recap your Sex and the City Match is: Carrie*

*A-List Match:* Lily Allen, Cameron Diaz, Drew Barrymore, Kate Hudson, Jamelia, Estelle, Agyness, Kirsten Dunst, Alesha Dixon, Sarah Harding.


## If you picked mostly C's  you're the Mysterious Flirt

*Signature flirt:*  You have an intriguing approach to flirting. You're that irresistible combination of awkward modesty which is offset by the wicked glint in your eye. A big part of your appeal is in your sexy modesty.

*Flirting style:* You're usually found standing quietly at the bar waiting for a drink, or letting your friends do most of the talking. You'll flash a secret smile here or there, and you love you drawing people in with your powerfully understated personality. You much prefer to listen than have all the attention. That's why you're such a mystery woman, and men love you for it.

*Famous for:* You always wait to be approached. Flirting might come relatively easy once you've been approached, but if the guy you like is equally aloof, or worse still, distracted by the throng of loud OTT girls giving him the eye, then you Miss Modest may go unnoticed.

*Deadly Weapon:* Killer eyes and secret smile.

*If you were a drink you'd be:* Black Velvet

*Movie Star from another time*: Ava Gardner

*Just to recap your A-list Match:* Shakira, Dita Von Teese, Kate Moss, Natalie Imbruglia, Scarlet Johansen, Keira Knightley, Uma Thurman, Daisy

Lowe, Sophie Ellis-Bexter, Penelope Cruz, Alexa Chung.

## If you picked mostly D's you're the Hard and Fast Flirt

***Signature flirt:*** In-your face sexuality. You're a vampy, trampy, foxy, feisty seductress and a total Sex Queen. You drip more sex appeal in your stiletto heel than most woman do in their whole outfit. You work those "come-hither, don't-dither" eyes, and guys can't get enough of your direct, sexed-up attitude – if they're not terrified that is!

***Flirting style:*** You're a woman with a capital W! You're an experimental, risk-taking sex bomb and Femme Fatale. You epitomise the "read my hips, not my lips" style of sex appeal.

***Qualities:*** You're quick with a smile, but you won't be seen dead making a fool of yourself, or being goofy – you tend to take yourself more seriously than that.

***Famous for:*** Oozing a modern day persona. Yours is a life made rich by sexy shenanigans.

***If you were a drink, you'd be:*** A Sex on the Beach.

***Movie star from another time:*** Mae West

***Just to recap your Sex and the City Match was:*** *Samantha*

***A-List Match:*** Lady Ga Ga, Madonna, Christine Aguilera, Rihanna, Sharon Stone, Paris Hilton.

## If you picked mostly E's you're the Tough Love Flirt

***Signature flirt:*** You know how to deliver with polish and poise when you want to, and equally you know how to exude a hint of "when I'm unleashed I'm a tiger" mystery. You can be cynical when it comes to men's intentions, but when you meet the right one – your barriers come tumbling down.

You're fearless and upfront. Once you've found someone you're attracted to you don't believe in wasting time.

*Flirting style*: You know the difference between assertive with aggressive. You watch for the signals and respond accordingly. You don't sulk and pout; you say what you mean and mean what you say.

*Famous for:* Being cool, calm and collected (and OTT when you need to be).

*Deadly weapon:* You're a sexual time-bomb waiting to go off.

*If you were a drink, you'd be*: A long, cool Vodka Tonic.

*Movie star from another time:* Katherine Hepburn

*Just to recap your Sex and the City Match was: Miranda*

*A-list Match:* Naomi Campbell, Janice Dickinson, Heather Mills, Pink, Tina Turner, Grace Jones, Courtney Love, Cher, Joan Jett, Katie Price, Angelina Jolie.


**Now**… I'm going to ask you to select the gestures you ticked from each of the above categories and list them below. This will help build your signature style. Simply pick the gestures that you're most comfortable with, or those you might use naturally anyway. The challenge is to build them into your flirt repertoire and use them on high rotation during each and every flirt session. Got that? If you're a real eager diva, you will select dozens and dozens and practice using them all, so you never run out of flirt ammo. Not ever!

As you get into the groove and find your feet, you'll see it starts to come naturally. And so the flirting dance begins. It really is that easy. Once you're in control of your killer moves, smiling your "special smile", whilst devouring his lips with your eyes, and flicking that hair like there's no tomorrow – he will cotton on to the fact that you're interested – believe me!

And before you can say, *ooh la la,* the two of you will be flirting your heads off. Right then, get that pen happening and list the moves you will bring into play each and every time you find yourself in a flirtatious situation.

***Which gestures will you use to knock ém dead with?***

1.

2.

3.

4.

5.

6.

7.

8.

9.

10.

*Now add in as many more as you like* ……………………………..

…………………………………………………………………………

…………………………………………………………………………

# DAY 2
## EYE CONTACT

Practice your eye-contact in the mirror, on friends or if you're feeling really brave, on random strangers!

### 1. The triangle gaze. Otherwise known as the "I could be interested in more than just coffee".

Often when we describe the *amazing* sensation of "looking into each other's eyes" we imagine direct, unblinking eye contact. But the most effective way of giving off the feeling of "looking longingly" is to change your focus from the left to the right pupil and hold for a maximum of five seconds each. Then, if you want to be really saucy, let your eyes wander down, and linger on his cheeks, his nose and finally come to rest, slap bang on his lips. Let your eyes hungrily devour his lips for another 5 seconds or so, then move your gaze slowly back up his face to his eyes, and alternate once again from left to right pupil. Phew. He'll soon know he's being manhandled! And if he doesn't get the feeling for what's on your mind soon, he's pretty thick!

### 2. The come-hither approach.

A smile says *a lot* about you. There are smirkers and half smilers and those who smile only with their mouths (we call them stingy smilers). But the genuine smile is impossible to miss, that's when the whole face lights up, the eyes crinkle, the cheeks rise – phwoar blimey – it's all happening! Practice a few different varieties so that when you unleash your smile, you know exactly what message you're putting out there. Develop a whole repertoire and practice – all day, everyday: confident, happy, pouty, sultry, flirty, foxy, wholesome, loving and of course, lustful! Learn hot to keep your smile fresh and topped up, even when you're in the middle of a

256

conversation. With a little bit of effort, you can manage a sublimely sexy look simply by being happy and smiley.

### 3. The Secret Smile

This is where you're smiling, but your eyes do all the work. Keep your mouth semi closed, let your cheeks reach right up to your eye-sockets and beam that love and happiness right out of your eyes – feel the luv! Throw in a head-tilt if you really want to knock him for a six. And then say something ridiculously fun like: *"I think the barmaid's got a crush on you"*.

Now you come up with some ideas of your own. It's OK if they're really silly. It's just to get you in the right frame of mind. And remember – it's meant to be fun!!

1.................................................................................

2.................................................................................

3.................................................................................

## *INTEGRATE FLIRTING INTO YOUR DAY-TO-DAY*

Get inside the Global Flirtzones and create your own personal flirt itinerary. Simply by activating your lifestyle changes, you will broaden your flirt-ortunities tenfold. Get the party started with a Flirt Squad cocktail bash and brainstorm new hotspots to hit. Just get out there and be a walking, talking, boozing, schmoozing, cruising Flirt Diva. Right now your answer to every invitation must be a resounding "Yes!" The more you place yourself in different social environments, the better you will get. And before long – perfecto! A wondrous Flirt Diva is born.

And think laterally – even the parks are brimming with flirting opportunities. Find an excuse to have a party in the park and get out there. It's just too easy to strike up a conversation with a hot dude *if* you've got the right props and you're the life of the party.

*Props:*

- Bite-size afternoon tea: cupcakes; scones and strawberries
- A bottle of bubbly and spare plastic glasses – no harm in offering a cute stranger a drink
- A dog to walk (borrow if necessary) and lap up the attention.
- An iPod  (Cue up a song and see if he can guess what it is)
- Bubble blowing liquid for big crazy bubbles
- A footy or cricket ball or bat – anything to do with sport will lure new friends
- A kite – anything they think they can do better than you will also work!
- Playing cards – someone might be up for a game of Snap!
- A book – always good if someone wants to ask "what you reading?"

# DAY 4

## PUT YOURSELF IN THE MAN-ZONE

One of the best ways to learn how men flirt is by watching them in action – funny that! Dip your toes in by going places where you can surreptitiously watch both men, and couples. Ideally you should make a date with a platonic mate to get in the right headspace to treat yourself to some man friendly activities. Play a game to "Spot the Flirt". Get down to a sports stadium, a racing track, or anywhere you will be able to observe men and the way they interact with each other, and of course with women.

Brush up on the "man signals" so you're clued up as to what to look out for. See for yourself which gestures are the most recognisable. Keep yourself hotwired on Man-Alert as much as possible. Become the expert on how to tell when a man is flirting, with you or anyone else for that matter!

Alternatively, head out to a busy area for an hour or so of "Couple Watching". Watch closely for the different signs and gestures between couples and see if you can tell who's in control. In other words, who's driving this flirt fest? See if you can pick up how couples mirror each other in a "monkey see, monkey do" kind of way. You'll notice that when they're standing and having a Special Moment, they'll lean in towards each other with their lower bodies facing each other – a term scientifically referred to as "crotch to crotch". It's a subtle and territorial means of showing the world they're together – and telling everyone to "back off!"

# DAY 5
## DEALING WITH REJECTION

If the fear of rejection is stopping you from moving forward, use this time to think about the issues *behind* the fear. What's really stopping you? If there is a deeper issue, stemming from a bad memory or experience, you really need to make the effort to get onto it. Revisit Step 1 and go through the relevant exercises and take action – whether that's reading in-depth about your issue or seeking professional help. The end result is simply that you will enjoy going out more, making a connection, and if it comes to it, making an approach. Sort out the obstacles that could be stopping you and work out for once and for all what you need to do to overcome your fear of rejection.

### *Or you could write an imaginary letter:*
Dear latest crush,

Thank you for your rejection of August 19. After careful consideration, I am happy to inform you that I gladly accept your rejection of me. These past few weeks I have been particularly fortunate in receiving an unusually large number of successes. With such a varied and promising field of suitors, it is now possible for me to accept the very few rejections I come by, yours included.

Despite your obvious previous experience in rejecting romantic applicants, I find that your rejection is proof that I am moving up in the world. Away from losers like you.

Best of luck in getting rejected yourself next time.

*Truthfully yours,* Aspiring Flirt Diva

## DAY 6

### SIGN UP FOR A DATING GAME

Once you've found a dating website that suits your personality and sounds like it might float your boat, it's absolutely worthwhile joining up. So long as you only use it in conjunction with other dating strategies – those which operate in The Real World! That means online dating must only ever take up a portion of your "personal time". It should never be the only outlet you use to snag a hot date.

Experiment with other events and activities as well, whether it's speed-dating, a book lovers club or a wine course for singles – just sign up, it's no biggie. Don't be one of those people who let all those things they "never did" build up. Ensure you've got flirt-ortunities galore.

Revisit Step 3 and go through the Action Diva suggestions. Act on your passions now, rather than sitting around saying "woulda, shoulda, coulda."

**Check out these tried and true dating sites:**
www.speeddater.co.uk
www.mysinglefriend.com
www.dating.guardian.co.uk
www.plentyoffish.com
www.matchmaker.com

**Or, for a taste of the bizarre. Or at the very least, for a giggle!**

*www.golddiggers.uk.com*
*www.fancyashag.com*
*www.sugardaddy.com*
*www.toyboywarehouse.co.uk*
*www.cheekybutlers.com*
*www.blackmaleescort.co.uk*
*www.elegance4her.com*

# DAY 7

## DIARY OF A FLIRT DIVA

*OK, Supergirl, quick spot-check to see how you've progressed so far…*

*Tick any of the following **if** they apply:*

1. *Have you been studying your female role models?*
2. *Signed up for any new challenges?*
3. *Done anything out of your comfort zone?*
4. *Gone out with platonic male friends to practise flirting?*
5. *Done any "couple watching"*
6. *Made any good eye contact with the opposite sex?*
7. *Flirted with anyone new?*

*If you ticked Yes! More than 4 times, you're on track. Yay you!*

If you ticked mainly No's, you're lagging behind. And I'm sorry but if you want the full Flirt Diva experience, you'll need to go back and refocus on the weak areas pronto. Well, no-one said this was going to be easy!!

## *Time for the Flirtabolical Do's & Don'ts*

### *Do:*

- Leave the house.

- Make eye contact.

- Get a Just-In-Case Wax.

- Have emergency ice-breaker tactics to hand.

- Watch and listen for the "signs".

- Tell goofy stories about yourself!

- Put yourself Out There.

- Be direct and ask questions.

- Flatter him senseless: "I think the barmaid's got a crush on you!"

- Laugh your head off at every joke.

- Engage your audience – you're here to entertain!

- Get out of your comfort zone.

- Breathe. Slow everything down, and drink less, not more!

- Wear fantastically sexy underwear.

- Keep open fluid body language.

- Be aware of your voice and how you're coming across.

- Sex up the tone and treat him to a very naughty smile.

## *But whatever you do, don't...*

- Wear lip-gloss that sticks to your hair when you do an almighty hair flick.

- End up flat on your face thanks to 6-inch heels.

- Hang around if the response isn't positive.

- Be fake (it'll be obvious from a mile away).

- Lose your dignity. Stay in control. Stay sober!

- Eat a big, sloppy curry before you step out.

- Nod encouragingly if you've got no idea what he's talking about, (it will be awkward if you're caught out).

- Put your make-up on with a trowel.

- Spend the whole conversation worrying about what *he's* thinking.

- Wear your big pants if you're going out for a big night.

- Go OTT with your gesturing and gyrating. Guys get intimidated when girls are too full on. Remember that!

### *Advanced Foolproof Tips*

SmileSmileSmileSmileSmileSmileSmileSmileSmileSmileSmileSmileSmile

## *Flirt Review: Creating your Flirt Profile*

Now that you've come to the end of Step-6, you should have a lot on your mind. Great! Write it down. But first, take a moment look back over your Flirt Diary to see how much you've accomplished since the beginning of this journey. Read back over your entries and consider the obstacles you've dealt with, and the challenges that are yet to come. Describe your new attitude, as well as the fears and insecurities that you've worked through along the way.

How are you feeling about yourself? This is all about you remember? What are you most proud of? Excited about? What can't you wait to try out? Don't be afraid to ask yourself the tough questions. How far have you come in getting on top of your issues? What is it that you still need to do? What is the one thing that is still holding you back from being the woman you know you can be? Make a pact to keep working on your issues. The self-work doesn't stop here – this is just the beginning.

Now head up a fresh page with the title Personalised Profile and complete each of the following sentences to find your Signature Style. You can elaborate as much as you like, using the material from the previous steps to jog your memory and give you an overall picture of your flirting personality – not just the person you are today, but the person you will grow into as you continue to practice and put all your new found knowledge into practice.

**Personalised Profile:**

My emotional state of mind is *i.e improving but still needs work!*

..........................................................................

My celebrity style is based on *i.e. Carry Bradshaw*

..........................................................................

If I was a movie star from another time I'd be *i.e Elizabeth Taylor*

..........................................................................

My action diva approach is *i.e to go for it! I'll try anything once.*

..........................................................................

My beauty style is *i.e Experimental*

...................................................... ................

My deadly weapon is *i.e my smile*

..........................................................................

My best quote is *i.e I like the way you think!*

..........................................................................

If I was a drink I'd be *i.e Long Island Iced Tea*

..........................................................................

My signature style is *i.e Cheeky Girly Flirt*

..........................................................................

# Congratulations you've completed your Step 6 missions!

*Step 6 Learning Outcomes*
*Key Points*

> ➤ Be sexually savvy about the signals you're putting out there.
>
> ➤ Approach with a smile and you're half way there.
>
> ➤ If he still doesn't get it after you've *hit him with your best shot,* ladies, you know the drill. Step away from the man!

*Checklist: The Flirt Diva's little bag of tricks*

- ✓ Name card (like a business card but with your personal details so no-one distracts you at work).
- ✓ Tic tacs/gum/mints
- ✓ Pencil/pen
- ✓ Digital cameral phone
- ✓ Note book
- ✓ Bullshit detector.

*Vamp Mantra:*

*I am Worthy!*

*I am Hot!*

*I am Queen of the Freakin' Universe!*

### *The Beginning of the Happy Ever After…*

So here we are the point of no return. There are no excuses now. You're armed and dangerous! You've come along way since the beginning of Operation Flirt and look at you now – you're a pro! You've sorted out your signature style, practiced your technique, you have your Flirt Squad in tow – now it's time to get out there to road-test your raunch and pull some full on Bond style flicks and dips.

Gone is li'l Miss Clueless, who once walked into a room full of good-looking blokes and freaked out the minute there was a Hot Man Alert. In her place is a killer vamp, oozing charisma, confidence and crackling conversation. You are in the words of Carrie Bradshaw "single and fabulous!" *Cheers!*

So what is it that makes the new you so alluring? Could it be as simple as being a Flirt Divafied version of your *old self*? The way you carry yourself and have a laugh at your own expense? The way you're ready to take a risk and roll the dice? Is it in your voice, your smile and the way your eyes glint and glisten, twinkle and listen?

It's all of these things and more! Who wouldn't want to hang-out with you? You're good. You're pornographically good! You've said goodbye to the insecurities, the doubts and all those traits that were holding you back. You're through with self-sabotage and tripping yourself up. You've lost the self-depreciation trip you were on – since it got you nowhere! And you're determined to quit mucking around and just go after what you want.

You feel weirdly level-headed and ready for any setbacks. You're shrewd enough to know it's not all going to be smooth sailing, but you've toughened up a lot during this process, and it's going to take more than one lousy rejection from sideshow Bob to hold you back. You're unstoppable now. You'll show them. You'll freaking well show all of them.

So here you are, raring to go, superstar of your own godamn flirt-festival. A fully divafied transmission vamp. Let's head out on to the field to sample some good-time *flirt, chat, rattle and roll!*

Picture this. It's 9.33pm. Your Friday night is in full swing at a crazy, sexy, cool bar. The vino is flowing, your conversation is sparkling, you feel good! You're fizzing with anticipation about the night ahead. This is your time. You've got a gazillion foolproof tips and puff-chatty pieces up your sleeve to let Freddy Fabulous know you fancy him. Now you just need to brace yourself for the frenzied scenes that will follow. And fear not, this Flirt Diva will be right behind you, cheering you on all the way.

Of course you'll have your Flirt-Squad in tow for moral support as well, so you won't have to worry about goofing up; and if you do, you know the drill, it's no biggie. Likewise, if you make a teensy mistake, don't sweat it. Soon you'll be shimmying and shaking your way through your signature moves. And before long – voila! You'll find yourself doing the *flirt cha-cha-cha* with Mr Omg! That's when you'll know how far you've come in your quest for Flirt Divadom – and how much more fun your life is because of it.

Now get out there and have the time of your life!

♥          ♥          ♥

## Welcome to the club!

If you would like some extra guidance in your quest for Flirt Divadom, I've created the Flirt Diva work-book and online community to share a download of the World's First Get Loved Up! Challenge. You'll find more step-by-step flirt tutorials and cheeky challenges. Where else would you find a master-class devoted to how to drip sexuality and get yourself in shape for the flirting Olympics? Just log onto www.flirtdiva.com

**JARGON BUSTER: *A flirt dictionary to help decipher the jargon***

1. Who is Flirtzilla?

*She's the crazy OTT chick; the one who will do **anything** to get her man. We're not here to be Flirtzilla! We have a little more class than that!*

2. What do you mean when you say, "don't be a crackwhore for love?"

*Don't give up your independence. Don't become addicted. Don't follow anyone around like a puppy. Just be yourself – and keep your own life!*

3. How do I perfect the come-hither look and not look like I've got a tic in my eye?

*Easy. You practice. In the mirror and with your Flirt-Squad. They can rate you how you're doing and give you feedback.*

4. What is an ICE?

*"In Case of Emergency". Think of it as an SOS, when you're with your gal pals and things are going really well with a guy – give them the ICE signal to let them know that this is NOT a good time to be interrupted!*

5. What is Flirophobia?

*It's when you're too chicken shit to flirt. This can be overcome. You could consider getting hypnotherapy for it, or you can simply practice. I think we know which is the smarter option...*

6. Why do I need to` micromanage' my sex appeal?

*Because as much as we like to think we can smoulder like sex demons if we really put our mind to it – it does take some effort. That's what Flirt Divas are all about. Managing the process of looking and feeling good.*

.

7.   What is a Triple S?

*A Triple S is a saucier, sexier, sassier version of you. It's an attitude that comes from within. And it has to be genuine. You can't fake it.*

8.  How do I know if I'm giving off the right "signals"?

*Are you smiling? Are you chatty? Are you interested? Then yes!*

9. Do I have good eye contact?

*Can you look someone in the eye without feeling weird and self-conscious? Then yes!*

10. What is OTT flirting?

*When you drunkenly insist he's coming back to yours even though he's hardly shown any interest!*

11. What is rejectaphobia?

*When you won't make an approach because the fear of rejection is too much for you. Time to get over that!*

12. How do I know if I'm scaring him off?

*He'll run!*

13. Flirtabolical do's and don'ts

*Your guide to what works and what's to be avoided at all costs.*


14. What are the Flirt Gang Rules?

*Keep it clean and don't play dirty.*


15. What are "slutastic traps"?

*These are a big no- no. They're used extensively by those otherwise known as come "prick-teases" and they're bad news.*


16. What is binge flirting?

*It's when you unleash a variety of the Pick 'n' Mix flirt gestures and bang that gorilla over the head with it.*


17. What is FAD (Flirt Anxiety Disorder)?

*It's when nerves get in your way and stop you from connecting with someone that you really like.*


18. What is a Point and Click tool?

*It's when you point your flirt radar towards someone and then make a gesture – either a wink, a wave or a smile.*


19. What is PMA – Positive Mental Attitude?

*It's your day to day outlook. Watch yours improve as you get your flirting mojo up to scratch.*

20. What's psycho-sexual self-survival?

*It's when you know how to protect yourself from getting hurt, (or just getting a bum deal from a very bad man!)*

21. What's emotional admin?

*It's when you sit down and get your emotional affairs in order.*

22. What's a flirt mojo?

*It's what you have when your confidence rises and you start flirting like there's no tomorrow.*

23. What's a flirt-onality?

*It's your full flirting personality revealed.*

24. What are flirt-ercises?

*It's what you do to kick-start your flirting prowess.*

25 What's the Flirt Diva vault?

*It's where your romantic history is stored away*

26. What are lust-busters?

*Lust busters are when you clam up because you like someone; or conversely when you go completely OTT and scare them away.*

28. What is Operation Take-Charge?

*It's when you do what needs to be done to smash free of your old life.*

29. What is a Flirt Squad?

*They're your wing-women and best friends – the girls' who will support and encourage you through your flirting journey.*

30. What is the flirts 'secret weapon?'

*It's her individuality – or what we call her 'signature style'. It's her smile, it's her eyes and the way she carries herself. It's what you'll have when you finish the 6-Step-plan!*

Lightning Source UK Ltd.
Milton Keynes UK
UKOW020838080513

210335UK00003B/130/P